Research Writing
in Dentistry

Research Writing in Dentistry

J. Anthony von Fraunhofer
MSc, PhD, C.Eng, C.Chem, C.Sci, FADM, FASM, FICorr, FRSC
Professor Emeritus
University of Maryland, Baltimore

WILEY-BLACKWELL

A John Wiley & Sons, Ltd., Publication

Edition first published 2010
© 2010 Blackwell Publishing

Blackwell Publishing was acquired by John Wiley & Sons in February 2007.
Blackwell's publishing program has been merged with Wiley's global Scientific,
Technical, and Medical business to form Wiley-Blackwell.

Editorial Office
2121 State Avenue, Ames, Iowa 50014-8300, USA

For details of our global editorial offices, for customer services, and for
information about how to apply for permission to reuse the copyright material in
this book, please see our website at www.wiley.com/wiley-blackwell.

Library of Congress Cataloging-in-Publication Data

Von Fraunhofer, J. A. (Joseph Anthony).
  Research writing in dentistry / J. Anthony von Fraunhofer. – 1st ed.
     p. ; cm.
  Includes bibliographical references and index.
  ISBN 978-0-8138-0762-1 (pbk.)
  1. Dentistry–Research–Methodology.   2. Technical writing   I. Title.
    [DNLM: 1. Dental Research–methods.   2. Writing.   3. Data Interpretation,
Statistical.   4. Research Design. WU 20.5 V945r 2010]
  RK80.V66 2010
  617.60072–dc22

                                                                    2009041426

A catalog record for this book is available from the U.S. Library of Congress.

Set in 10/12pt Palatino by Aptara® Inc., New Delhi, India

1   2010

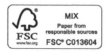

MIX
Paper from
responsible sources
FSC   FSC® C013604
www.fsc.org

This book is dedicated to past, present and future dental researchers. Dentistry as we know it would be impossible without you.

Contents

Preface

The purpose of this book is to provide the inexperienced scientist, notably junior faculty, residents, and predoctoral clinical students, with practical guidance on how to go about finding a research project and how to design appropriate studies and then write up the results. In order to provide a useful "how to" book, the approach is to give concrete advice and information as well as show how a program of research work can be developed, analyzed, and presented.

It order to complete a research project and write it up as a thesis or dissertation, a publication in a scientific paper or a presentation at a scientific meeting, the generated data must be subjected to statistical analysis. Accordingly, Part II of this book covers statistics and statistical analysis. The treatment is based in large part upon the Microsoft Excel spreadsheet and the ProStat statistical program using practical examples.

I thank my daughter, Dr. Nicola von Fraunhofer, and my good friends and respected colleagues, Dr. Sharon Siegel, Dr. Leslie Gartner, and Dr. Sean Wetterer, for reading and commenting upon various chapters. Their advice, comments, and suggestions have been invaluable. On a personal note, I like to express my appreciation to my wife Susan for her patience, support, and generous TLC during the writing of this book.

J. Anthony von Fraunhofer

Part I
Organizing, Writing, and Performing Dental Research

Introduction

Academics commonly are required to do research and publish to achieve promotion and tenure. Undertaking a research project is also an increasingly common course requirement for undergraduate and professional school students. Admission into good colleges and universities often necessitates that prospective students demonstrate intellectual achievement above and beyond good grades, and this frequently requires some form of research endeavor or at least participation in a research project. Similar considerations are equally applicable for new graduates or senior year predoctoral students who are attempting to gain admittance into graduate programs. Without some form of research credentialing, graduate program directors may pass over viable candidates in favor of a person who has gone that extra yard during predoctoral training. In other words, it is very beneficial to one's career prospects to be able to demonstrate intellectual curiosity through some sort of research involvement.

Most people, however, are immediately intimidated when confronted with the prospect of doing research and there tend to be feelings of "I am too old, tired, inexperienced, undereducated or too busy to do research." Such attitudes, though common, are a disservice to the prospective researcher in particular and to the advancement of knowledge in general. Further, such attitudes deprive the putative researcher of the pleasure and satisfaction of discovery and the chance to do something that no one else has ever done before. We all know the pleasurable feeling (and, let us face it, the slight feeling of superiority) that one gets from the simple task of sharing knowledge or expertise with someone else. "Hey, I've found a good short cut to the supermarket/office/mall etc." or "Have you tried this?" are very common and simple demonstrations of time well spent in acquiring new knowledge ... and that really is what research is all about.

The approach adopted in the following chapters has been to identify an issue that needs to be resolved and show how this can lead to a series of

3

research projects. Then, the suggested research projects will be outlined to indicate how the projects should be pursued.

This book provides a practical guide to performing a research project and, equally important, how to share that knowledge with other people be it in the form of a thesis/dissertation, a scientific paper, a poster or an oral presentation such as a lecture. To all intents and purposes, research data that are not shared with others do not exist but, as virtually every graduate student will tell you, communicating that information is difficult. Most of us know one or more people who are "ABD" (all but dissertation), people who cannot complete their master's or PhD degrees because they have yet to write up their research findings as a thesis or dissertation. Consequently, the second objective of this book is to help undergraduate and postgraduate students and other knowledge generators to write up their research and gain the recognition that their hard work and efforts truly deserve.

What Is Research?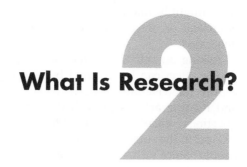

Dictionaries typically define research as:

a. A diligent search or inquiry, or
b. A scientific investigation and study to discover facts

A moment's reflection tells us that everyone does some form of research virtually every day of their lives. The actual task might be as simple as locating the nearest veterinary practice when one moves into a new neighborhood, finding a new physician or dentist, locating a supermarket or simply checking street maps to find the fastest and most convenient route to work each day. Research may also involve far more complex undertakings such as investigating the role of zinc in preventing prostate cancer or the causes of metal allergy in patients with metallic dental restorations. In other words, any intellectual undertaking that involves asking, and answering, questions that require the questioner to acquire new knowledge or organizing existing knowledge to answer questions is, by definition, research.

FINDING A RESEARCH PROJECT

Research in the academic setting is the generation and/or acquisition of new knowledge but in order to assure success in a research project, there has to be an underlying interest in the subject on the part of the researcher. The researcher must find a field or area of interest and then decide upon a specific question or problem that has to be answered or explained. Even if one's research activity involves simply helping a senior researcher in his or her work or doing rote experiments under the direction of someone else within the scope of a larger study, you can still make a contribution to advancing knowledge by asking why something happens or whether there might be another way to perform the same task. Ask; if the answer is unclear or unsatisfactory, look into the matter. That is how ideas are generated.

Asking oneself why something happens the way it does or if a particular effect can be avoided by a change in material selection or procedure likewise are fertile fields for projects. Looking at the literature and reading articles published in different journals also raise research questions—clearly, if you read the article, then you obviously have some interest in the subject, so why not take the next step and look into it more deeply? Since virtually no research paper is definitive and, therefore, cannot satisfy all aspects of a problem, a careful review of the literature will soon raise a number of questions worth investigating.

There are several interpretations of the literature on a particular topic. It is possible, for example, that what is not said is more important than what is said. It is very rare for any published paper or even a textbook to cover every aspect of any given subject and, for example, let us not forget that Einstein's relativity theory did not address what happens when a particle exceeds the speed of light. Thus, what has not been covered in a published paper or research program offers fertile ground for further research by others.

Similarly, a technique may have been used in a particular study not because it was the best approach but because it was the only one available to the researchers. Many important research projects and experimental findings have evolved from asking such simple questions as "why did someone use this particular approach or technique rather than something else?"

Simply put, all research can be summed up as shown in Table 2.1.

At the start of the project, the researcher must formulate a theory or supposition and this is known as a *hypothesis*. The hypothesis is the basis or framework for the research since the program of work is directed at establishing the validity of the hypothesis.

Most clinicians actually formulate a hypothesis every time they see and treat a patient. For example, a patient may present with complete denture and complain of irritated cracks and fissures at the corner of the mouth, and possibly excess saliva. The immediate diagnosis is that the patient is

Table 2.1 Basics of research.

What are you going to do?
How are you going to do it?
What do you expect to find?
What are you going to do with the information?

suffering from angular cheilitis caused by loss of vertical dimension. This would be the basic hypothesis or H_0. The alternative hypothesis, H_1, is that the cheilitis is the result of a vitamin B deficiency or a yeast infection (e.g., a candida-induced stomatitis). Thus, when the clinician examines the patient and finds that the occlusion is balanced and that the patient has not lost vertical dimension, he or she will likely decide that H_0 has not been validated or proved. The clinician then will reject H_0 and accept the alternative hypothesis, H_1, and treat the patient accordingly, that is, prescribe vitamin supplementation and/or attempt to eliminate the yeast infection. In other words, when a clinician evaluates a patient and decides upon a course of treatment, the thought process parallels that of a researcher deciding upon a project, developing basic and alternative hypotheses and then working to validate or reject the hypotheses.

Although deciding upon a suitable research project and formulating a hypothesis may appear to be daunting, in fact, neither task is difficult as long as you maintain an open, receptive mind. The latter permits you, the researcher, an opportunity to ask questions that have not already been answered in detail by others. However, you the researcher must always adhere to the basic principle that if you are not interested in the subject, then doing research can become very tedious and might even be abandoned if the experience becomes too unpleasant.

Four things must be borne in mind with regard to research:

1. No one, repeat no one, walks into the laboratory first thing in the morning, shakes a test tube, shouts "Eureka" and writes off to the Nobel Prize Committee! Most of the time, one looks at data readings, charts, and graphs and then mutters darkly about the need to repeat measurements or even go back to the drawing board because things did not work out as expected.

2. It cannot be stressed enough that the first and most essential task before starting any research project is to review the literature. The literature will tell you what has been done, how it was done, and usually what it all means. Although reviewing the literature was mentioned earlier, it is worth repeating that every hour spent online or in the library will save at least 10 or more hours in the laboratory.

3. Focus on the view, not the window. Novel techniques and sophisticated laboratory instrumentation are often wonderful advances, but focusing on the methodology rather than on what you are actually trying to investigate more often than not leads to frustration and disappointment.

4. If it does not make sense, it is probably wrong. Weird and totally unexpected things do happen and are real phenomena but most of the time, things that are wildly different from the norm are usually

artifacts. This is why all experiments have to be repeated several times and, indeed, all the experimental parameters including the test materials have to be checked just to make sure that the untoward observation was not simply another example of the law of universal cussedness. (If things can go wrong, they will.)

Research Planning

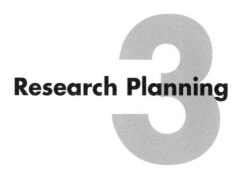

Einstein once said, "If we knew what we doing, we would not call it research." However, we can level the playing field. Seneca the Younger stated "Luck is what happens when preparation meets opportunity" and Louis Pasteur paraphrased this as "Fortune favors the prepared mind." All great philosophers, generals, artists, writers, and creative people make careful preparations before embarking upon any endeavor. If thorough preparation is good enough for the greatest of minds, then it is mandatory for the rest of us.

Ideally, before starting upon the research project, the researcher must formulate a theory or supposition and this is known as a *hypothesis*. The hypothesis is the basis or framework for the research since the research program is directed at establishing the validity of the hypothesis. This process is outlined in Figure 3.1.

Unfortunately, developing the research hypothesis in a clear and methodical manner, as shown in Figure 3.1, is not always possible and establishing a basic hypothesis is often very difficult. If the researcher is working toward a higher degree, then it is sensible to seek the advice of a supervisor or mentor for guidance in developing a research project. When the researcher does not have access to a suitable supervisor, then the research hypothesis must be formulated through careful and critical appraisal of the literature.

In many cases it may not be possible to formulate a research hypothesis before starting on the research program. For example, a dental material or drug can be studied without formulating a working hypothesis at the outset, a typical case being a study directed at evaluating or characterizing the properties of the new product. Once the initial work has been completed, the researcher can then undertake research aimed at explaining the behavior or properties of the material in question, that is, to formulate a working hypothesis. Similar considerations apply in a wide variety of projects; that is, the researcher performs a few initial or exploratory

9

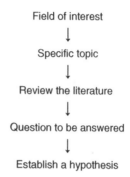

Field of interest

↓

Specific topic

↓

Review the literature

↓

Question to be answered

↓

Establish a hypothesis

Figure 3.1 Developing the research hypothesis.

experiments that provide a "feel" for the subject. Then, based on the findings of the initial work, it is possible to develop the working hypothesis and get started on the full program of work.

Another approach to developing a hypothesis and research program is to apply a new technique to an old problem, that is, a re-research project. While useful data may often be produced by this type of study, it is possible that the researcher could be criticized for examining a nonproblem, that is, the focus is on the window not the view. Common sense should be the guide here. If the research produces facts and figures in place of previously vague generalizations, then the work is valuable. But if the project is directed at doing yet another study of an old and well-known phenomenon using a new technique but which has little likelihood of generating new knowledge, then the research project might be ill-advised.

PLANNING THE RESEARCH PROJECT

There is no set approach to any problem. Individuals will tackle tasks in completely different ways, and this includes such common activities as driving or painting a house as well as more complex undertakings such as research planning and experimentation. Consequently, it is only possible to advise and recommend rather than to lay down rigid guidelines on how to do research. The ideal approach is indicated in Figure 3.2 and can be summarized as follows:

a. Project is established with a (working) research hypothesis
b. The literature is critically reviewed—if the subject has already been studied in depth, then the project must be changed or modified

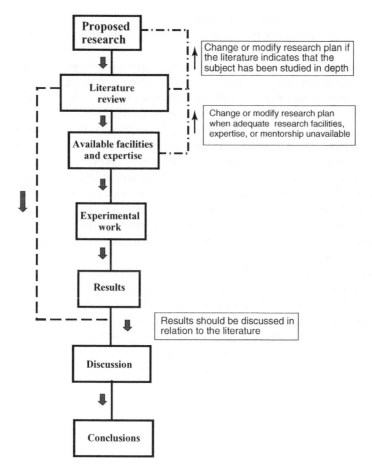

Figure 3.2 The ideal research project. *Note*: If the findings of the study differ markedly from those of previous studies, secondary experiments should be performed to determine the source of these differences and to ensure that the findings of the study are valid.

c. Laboratory facilities, availability of materials, and, notably, advice and mentorship (guidance) should be evaluated and secured—if suitable facilities, mentoring, or equipment is not available, then the project should be changed or modified
d. The experimental work is performed
e. Results are evaluated and subjected to statistical analysis
f. The results are discussed and the findings related to the previously reported data in the literature
g. Conclusions are drawn

A new class of material or drug, an improved testing methodology, a change in test parameters, and a host of other factors can and usually will make your own work unique and special.

There are, however, two highly important factors in research. First, there is intuition. The experienced and, as often as not, the inexperienced researcher will feel that something does not appear to be "right" or that the findings are not in accord with the anticipated results. When this happens, the good researcher will return to his or her study and look for any sources of error or unexpected variability before deciding that the observed findings are real rather than artifact. A second factor that enters into research is the basic principle that it is virtually impossible to prove a negative. Proving that a treatment plan, clinical procedure, or a new material or drug is beneficial to the patient is generally straightforward. Likewise, harmful or adverse effects upon the patient are usually unequivocal. However, to prove that something is not harmful is extremely difficult, if not impossible.

Researchers must develop a critical sense. It is important to remember that even though a paper might have been published in a good journal by a reputable author, it does not automatically mean that the findings are correct or that they have been interpreted correctly. If the discussion and conclusions of a published paper are not in accord with the experimental results, or when several authors hold differing opinions on the same phenomenon, there is scope for re-examination.

Performing Research

In the same way that people rarely perform the same task in identical ways, every researcher has an individual approach to tackling a research project. Nevertheless, there are three principal approaches to research once the basic hypothesis has been established:

1. *Trial-and-error approach*: Random experiments are performed until a promising line of research is found. The researcher then determines which factor produced the required result or the greatest effect and proceeds to work in ever-widening circles about this central point.
2. *Progressive approach*: There is a methodical progression from some point at which every parameter is fixed to another point with each parameter being varied in turn (while every other parameter is kept constant) until all variables have been evaluated. This process is repeated until the desired end point has been reached although careful use of statistics can simplify the research methodology. Interesting sidelines or offshoots of the main program are followed up only after the major pattern has been established and fully investigated.
3. *Direct approach*: The project follows a rapid and direct progression from a starting point, which is well established and quantified, to the desired end product, with minor excursions along any interesting sidelines.

None of these approaches is completely satisfactory and two or three of them may be combined within a single project. Although it is important that the approach is always directed toward accepting or rejecting the null hypothesis (H_0), other pressures may affect the researcher's strategy. Many younger researchers are pushed by their mentors, departmental chairperson or management to publish their findings as soon as possible, the so-called "publication fever." While early and frequent publication may satisfy such demands, it is easy to overlook significant findings in

13

one's haste to publish. In contrast, the slow pedantic approach is almost guaranteed to be successful but can be tedious and it usually takes much longer to achieve publishable results.

The author prefers to carry out a few preliminary experiments or pilot studies to determine which approach to adopt. This involves fixing all the experimental parameters and running an initial trial. Then the most important parameter is varied and the experiment repeated. If this trial is successful, a series of experiments is planned and then performed and directed toward the desired results, but all the variables are noted down and a record of any promising offshoots is kept. If the intuitive or reasoned result is confirmed experimentally, ancillary experiments are performed which will prove or disprove the major finding. Then one's steps must be retraced and all the results and findings checked to ensure that the reasoning used is valid and that every experiment is repeatable. The null hypothesis may then be accepted. At this stage it is possible to follow up the interesting sidelines that might have been revealed during the course of the investigation.

There are, however, two situations that can develop. First, the major approach may not be successful and therefore a sideline might have to be followed before any progress is made. Second, the sideline may be irrelevant to the aim of the investigation but can be more interesting and important than the major project and a new hypothesis may then be established. In either case it is better to proceed in a direct line from the starting point to the desired conclusion, even if the research is unsuccessful, than to investigate every interesting sideline. Attempts to study every small factor can waste several years before any progress is made.

The author also likes to write up research reports (or even papers) at regular intervals, for example every 2–3 months, as the research progresses. This has the advantage that the research program is under continuous review and also the relevance of interesting sidelines is often demonstrated. If the intention is to obtain a higher degree, writing the thesis can then become simply collating the research reports and papers into a unified appraisal of the overall study.

RESEARCH EQUIPMENT

The materials and methods involved in the research project must be standardized as far as possible. Measuring gauges, balances, and analytical techniques should be regularly checked against standards. This, of course, is not always possible in clinical work but careful consideration of factors such as oral hygiene, general health, oral and general pathology, patient cooperation, and psychological involvement may avoid complications both in the early stages and later on as the study progresses.

The assumption so far has been that the researcher is involved in an *in vitro* or laboratory-based study. In general, these laboratory or "benchtop" studies are a lot easier and more straightforward than clinical studies for a number of reasons. Clinical studies, particularly those involving human subjects, are fraught with difficulties because of the multiplicity of inherent variables and the problems associated with patient follow-up after treatment.

Ideally, the study will yield quantifiable data such as changes in physical properties or strength, blood chemistry, enzymes and other biochemical markers, etc. Such data can be readily subjected to statistical analysis using parametric methods (see Part II).

The researcher must keep accurate records and every experiment should be performed under controlled conditions and as accurately as possible, with only one parameter being varied at a time. A single or "one off" test is rarely acceptable and every experiment should be performed several times to ensure reproducibility and both the accuracy and validity of the obtained data.

Each phase of the research program should be finalized as far as possible. What this means is that all calculations, determinations, and statistical analyses should be performed before moving on to the next phase. If the statistical analyses indicate inconclusive data, perform additional studies to increase the sample population and provide a better basis for statistical comparisons.

At every stage in an investigation, however, the researcher should reappraise both the latest work that has been completed and previous studies to ensure that the overall program is on track and that a coherent, interrelated body of work is being accumulated. These are general but useful rules to follow and adherence to them can obviate considerable repetition of work by ensuring that the amassed data will permit acceptance or rejection of the null hypothesis.

EXPERIMENTAL METHODS

In recent years several trends have become apparent in science, academia, and industry. These include the increasing sophistication of science and scientists, the explosion in computer technology, the incredible informational resource of the internet and the intense competition between scientific journals to publish the highest quality papers and articles. As a result, journal editors, editorial review boards, thesis committees, department chairmen, and so forth place greater demands upon the researcher and the research project, thesis, and published paper. Any published paper or thesis is now subjected to intense and critical review before acceptance and the reviewer always looks for certain key components and expects the researcher to address most, if not all, of the following questions:

1. Is the problem defined and can a working hypothesis be established?
2. Which parameters exert the greatest influence on the system to be studied?
3. What appears to be the best approach to studying the problem?
4. Is the test method reliable and accurate?
5. What statistical tests should be performed to analyze the data?
6. How many samples (specimens) are needed to achieve statistically meaningful data?
7. Has there been a satisfactory review of the literature?

It follows, therefore, that once a project has been selected, the experimental method or testing technique must be decided upon. If the literature indicates several alternative test methods or procedures, adopt the one that is the most straightforward or the one that fits with your own abilities and the available research facilities and equipment. It is also necessary to decide whether accelerated test methods are justified or necessary in laboratory studies, if double-blind procedures should be used in clinical trials, and also to check whether the test method or procedure will introduce any perturbation of the system. The latter is a very important consideration in both clinical and laboratory studies since the test method can sometimes affect the observed results and lead to incorrect conclusions.

Statistical analysis has been mentioned above and the need for proper statistical evaluation of the research data cannot be overemphasized. If you do not have a sound background in statistics, consult a statistician. It is almost impossible to get a paper published in a good journal without adequate statistical analysis of the data. Fortunately, most computer spreadsheet programs such as Microsoft Excel have excellent statistical analysis capabilities built into them and more advanced analyses can be performed with a variety of readily available computer programs.

Laboratory studies tests generate numerical data, for example, material strength values, solubilities, changes in biochemical markers, etc, and these can be evaluated relatively easily by parametric methods. The latter include analysis of variance with follow-up procedures such as the Duncan, Scheffé, and Tukey HSD (honestly significant difference) tests to determine differences between mean values or between groups of data. Nonparametric data are information that has been rated rather than precisely measured, for example, degree of inflammation, pain levels and so forth, and these require rather different statistical analyses, known as nonparametric testing. Nonparametric analyses include the Mann–Whitney U test, the Wilcoxon matched-pairs test, and the Spearman's rank correlation coefficient. Deciding upon the appropriate statistical test and the necessary sample size for adequate data analysis is difficult without the help of a good statistician but can be done by consulting any one of a number of readily available statistics books or computer-based programs.

CONCLUSIONS

There is no such thing as the perfect experiment, the ideal technique, or the infallible research worker. We all make mistakes but our capabilities and expertise are improved when we recognize and learn from the inevitable errors and miscalculations that occur in every research project. Critical appraisal and constant review of research work, both by ourselves as well as by trusted and knowledgeable friends and colleagues, will ensure that the research program makes logical, forward progress.

It is okay, if not inevitable, to make mistakes. Making the same mistake repeatedly, however, is not acceptable. Always double check each and every calculation and look at the findings to check that they make sense. A misplaced decimal point or using the wrong units can make nonsense of any study. Even the mighty NASA program makes silly mistakes as shown by the satellite that went awry because somebody forgot to convert feet and inches to metric distances.

Research can and should be fun. There is an immense satisfaction in generating new knowledge and to revising and building upon established, but often incorrect, information. As long as one can ask "Why?" and then try to answer the question, one's personal growth and development will continue throughout life.

How to Design a Research Study

Let us suppose that a colleague has come to you with an interesting observation. She noticed that there appeared to be marked differences in cutting performance of burs from two different manufacturers (Figure 5.1). Since Bur A costs about 50% more than Bur B, but cuts more efficiently and for longer, should she recommend changing the bur supplier?

Based on her observations, Bur A (from Dentburs Inc.) appears to show a progressive decrease in cutting performance with increased cutting time. In contrast, Bur B (from United Burs Inc.) initially showed good performance, identical to that of Bur A, for up to 4 minutes but then there was a dramatic drop in performance from 4 to 5 minutes. Thereafter, the cutting rate continued to drop to an unacceptable level at 8 minutes.

INITIAL ANALYSIS

Bur A showed a progressive loss in cutting efficiency, presumably as the bur wore down in use. The wear was uniform and progressive during use so that the cutting efficiency decreased at a steady but predictable rate.

Bur B showed a sudden drop in efficiency after a short time (4 minutes) of cutting. The marked change in performance could be due to accelerated wear, loss of abrasive or some other effect that prevented the bur from performing in a predictable and satisfactory manner.

The data indicate that although Bur A costs more, it lasts longer. Clearly there is something different between the two burs but what and why?

If this question was simply an interaction or passing comment between colleagues at a social gathering or between partners in a 2–3 person dental practice, one might simply buy a few burs from the two companies and try them out. The stakes, however, become much larger if one has to consider the purchase of thousands of dental burs each year for a large dental clinic, a dental school or a military base, particularly if the purchasing or

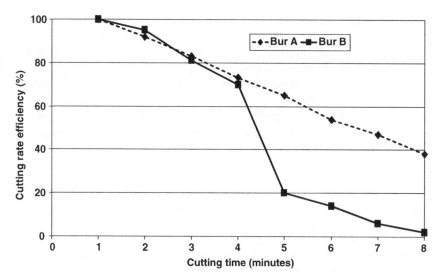

Figure 5.1 Cutting performances of burs from different manufacturers.

procurement officer is reluctant (or cannot) buy some burs from one man-ufacturer, and then has to approach another company for other burs etc. Now, you are facing the question of whether all burs of all types should be purchased from *Dentburs Inc.* or *United Burs Inc.* with the decision being based upon a single data set, with annual expenditures of thousands of dollars at stake.

QUESTIONS

Before even considering all the ramifications, certain issues need to be ad-dressed regarding your colleague's comments on Bur A and Bur B before any decision can be made with regard to bulk purchases of all dental burs. The first question is whether there is really a difference between Bur A from *Dentburs* and Bur B from *United Burs*, and this should be addressed as follows:
1. How was cutting efficiency measured?
    a. Was it based on clinical impressions or were actual quantifiable mea-surements made?
2. Were the burs of the same type?
    a. Were the burs identical in design and fabricated from the same ma-terial (i.e., were they either carbide burs or diamonds and did they have the same dimensions, number of blades, grit size, etc.)?
3. Were the cutting conditions the same for both burs?

    a. Were both burs used in the same handpiece at the same rotational speed and the same coolant flow rate to cut the same substrate?

    b. Was the applied load (the downward pressure on the handpiece) the same for both burs throughout testing?

    c. Were the cutting studies performed on teeth or an artificial but reproducible substrate?

4. Were the cutting studies performed with only one bur from each manufacturer or were several burs tested and the cutting efficiencies averaged?

5. Were the burs cleaned or sterilized between cuts?

Let us assume that all the cutting conditions were identical, a number of burs of each type were tested and quantifiable measurements were made (e.g., an assistant timed the sectioning of intact and caries-free adult molar teeth with six burs of each type). Although averages were calculated, no statistics were performed because the sample size was small or because statistical software was unavailable. Give the above, one now has to ask certain questions specific to your colleague's observations:

1. Is there a real difference between the two burs or were the data simply artifact?

2. Were the tested burs typical for that type of bur from each manufacturer or is there a batch variation for Bur A, Bur B, or both?

3. Is the observed behavior of Bur A typical of all burs manufactured by *Dentburs Inc.*?

4. Is the observed behavior of Bur B typical of all burs manufactured by *United Burs Inc.*?

5. Which behavior (that of Bur A or Bur B) is the norm for burs of the same design manufactured of the same materials by other companies?

6. How well do Bur A and Bur B perform compared to comparable burs from other manufacturers?

7. What controls should be used?

By now, it is obvious that we are no longer dealing with the simple issue of whether a single type of bur from an individual manufacturer is possibly better but more expensive than the same type of bur from another manufacturer. Instead, we are dealing with quality control and quality assurance (QC/QA) issues for products from two companies as well as the underlying question of what we want from any dental bur and for how long and at what cost. Suddenly, we have gone from buying a few burs and trying them for a couple of days to having to make major decisions with numerous ramifications.

Just what should we do and how do we do it? Let us break down the problem into components that can be addressed separately even though we want to have a coherent and hopefully comprehensive study.

Cutting conditions

1. Fabricate or purchase a standardized test system. The test system should mimic dental cutting on teeth or artificial substrates in a reproducible and quantifiable manner so that multiple burs can be tested under the same conditions. The system should also allow different handpieces to be tested.
2. Decide upon a single type of handpiece with a reproducible and controlled speed (bur rotational speed) and a controlled water coolant flow rate.

    Factors: Bur rotational speed affects cutting rate; coolant flow rate affects cutting rate; coolant spray pattern affects cutting rate.
3. Decide upon the cutting regimen and duration of cutting time.

    Factors: Applied cutting load; continuous cutting for a predetermined time or a succession of cuts of finite duration; length of cut (whether the full or a partial length of the bur is used for cutting).
4. Decide upon cutting substrate. Teeth are biological materials that are inherently variable in properties and dimensions, and can be difficult to obtain for test purposes. Artificial substrates are convenient, reproducible in properties and cutting data are quantifiable but do they accurately mimic the properties of dental hard tissue?

    Factors: Characteristics of the cutting substrate; thickness of the substrate (relates to length of cut).

Materials and methods (experimental details)

1. *Test equipment*: Clearly you need some type of quantifiable testing system that can hold the handpiece and bur and apply it under a known load to the cutting sample at a known rate. If such a system is not already available to you, then perusal of the literature will provide several suitable designs which can be fabricated.
2. *Test methodology*:
    a. Again, the literature will provide details on how other cutting studies were performed and the cutting substrate used in those studies. Following their lead immediately provides your work with an accepted (i.e., previously published) methodology and avoids the need for you to develop a testing regimen yourself. In the present cutting study project, using an applied load of 100 g mimics the average pressure that a restorative dentist uses in practice while much

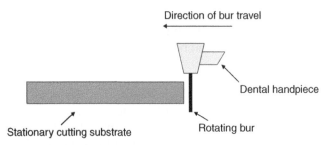

Figure 5.2 Arrangement of cutting substrate and bur positioning in cutting studies.

higher loads (300 g or higher) are common for oral surgeons when resecting teeth. Likewise, feather-light loads might be used for polishing but might not be appropriate for cavity preparations.

b. The test load on the handpiece that you select should be geared to the intended application of the bur you are studying and the audience you wish to reach. Restorative dentists have different operating parameters from oral surgeons, etc. Such considerations will dictate the precise methodology you adopt.

c. Another factor would be the length of cut the bur is expected to perform (Figure 5.2) and generally the length of substrate cut should be the same or shorter than that of the bur.

Quite different cutting data may be found with different substrate–bur arrangements (Figure 5.3).

Accordingly, the orientation of the cutting instrument (the bur), the dental handpiece and the cutting substrate should be arranged

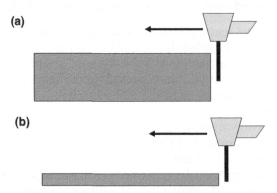

Figure 5.3 Bur–substrate arrangements: The bur may be shielded from coolant spray in schema (a) whereas only the bur tip is used for cutting in schema (b).

to avoid "end" effects and shielded (i.e., closed) as opposed to open access cutting.

3. *Measurements*:
   a. The rule here is that what you measure and how you measure it often dictates the findings. Adopting previously published measurement parameters is obviously sensible but blind acceptance is not always advisable. Cutting efficiency or cutting rate studies can involve weight change of the test substrate, time to transect a known distance of material, change in required force as well as various other approaches. The one you adopt can be specific to you but the derived data should always be in a form that allows you to obtain reproducible data and enables you to compare your data with those of other workers. In the example shown in Figure 5.1, Bur A was compared with Bur B in terms of cutting efficiency. However, no information was provided on what was measured, how it was measured, or even what "cutting efficiency" actually means. In other words, the information is largely meaningless in terms of quantifiable data.
   b. Another factor, in the present case of cutting studies, is how long a bur should be used, that is, how many cuts is a realistic evaluation of bur performance? Expecting a bur to cut a hard material such as tooth enamel continuously for 20 minutes when that bur costs only $1 may be expecting too much, particularly if cutting performance decreases sharply after 1–2 minutes. If the bur cutting rate decreases sharply after a few minutes, the dentist will find it more economical to switch to a new bur than to continue working with a poorly performing bur. Therefore, extended duration cutting studies might be unrealistic for certain types of cutting instrument.
   c. In a study like the present case, cutting could be evaluated in 30-second increments with each evaluation being performed until a predetermined end point is reached, for example, an unacceptable cutting rate under the adopted test conditions.
4. *Tests to be performed*: Now that we have a suitable testing system in place and we know how we can perform the requisite testing, a large number of different tests can be undertaken. The planned testing will determine what specimens we need. The following indicate the wide range of testing that can be performed but a note of caution must be sounded—a single researcher cannot investigate every aspect of a program of work unless the studies are prioritized. Possible priorities are suggested by the ordering of the following studies.
   a. Intra-bur studies, for example, would indicate the average performance of Type A, Type B, and any other burs over a regimen of ten 30-second cuts. Such tests would characterize the performance of

each type of bur. The data would indicate the inherent variability within the performance of a given type of bur over a certain number of cuts as well as indicate the operating life (i.e., durability) of that bur.

b. Inter-bur studies would compare the performance of Type A versus Type B burs, etc. Comparisons could be made between different burs at the start of cutting, after five cuts and after ten cuts. This permits comparison of bur durability and cutting longevity.

c. The effect of handpiece load on cutting efficiency of any type of bur can be evaluated as can the effect of lighter or heavier loads on relative performances. Cutting performances of different burs under the same range of loads also can be evaluated.

d. The effect of water coolant flow rates on cutting efficiency of any given type of bur can be evaluated as can interactive effects between coolant flow rate and applied load on cutting efficiency. Likewise, cutting performances of different burs under different flow rates can be evaluated and compared.

e. Improvements in cutting performance from chemical modification of the coolant water (chemomechanical effects) can also be studied for different burs and, indeed, for different cutting substrates.

f. Intra-bur and inter-bur comparative differences in cutting performance of burs that are used on a variety of substrates, for example, metals, composite resins, and dental amalgam. The interactive effects of cutting substrate change and cutting performance can also be evaluated for different burs under different applied loads, coolant flow rates, and chemomechanical effects.

It should be apparent from the above that a very large number of studies that will yield potentially useful data are possible using a single test system. Further, all of these tests have evolved from one fairly simple example and the associated question of whether one bur is better than another. The limitation here is that of one's imagination and curiosity. However, one should not undertake a large number of studies on an uncommon or rarely used type of bur, for example, unless there are good grounds for doing so. The rule of thumb should always be to go from the general to the specific when one is starting out.

5. *Test materials*: In the present example, two aspects have to be decided upon, namely the cutting substrate and the cutting instruments (burs) to be evaluated.

a. In the initial (pilot) stage, only one cutting substrate should be selected. Additional materials can be studied once a body of data has been assembled regarding cutting instrument performance for a given substrate.

b. There are numerous bur manufacturers and a vast number of different types of burs. It is not possible, in one lifetime, to study every bur from every manufacturer. Accordingly, intra-bur studies should be undertaken with common or representative burs from several but not all manufacturers in order to limit the number of studies that are performed. Inter-bur studies should be limited with regard to the numbers of bur types that are investigated.

c. While one might question whether, for example, a diamond bur might be better than a carbide bur, the determining factor will be the cutting substrate. A number of studies have already shown that one class of bur (e.g., diamonds) is preferred for cutting brittle materials such as dental enamel while another class (e.g., carbides) is more suitable for ductile materials such as dentin and cementum. Factors such as these should also be considered when planning a research project and, as always, consulting the literature will ensure that appropriate and relevant testing will be performed.

d. The number of burs tested in each segment of the study is important if statistical analysis is to be performed, and bearing in mind that statistical testing is virtually mandatory for any thesis, dissertation or published paper. Pilot studies can be performed in duplicate or triplicate but large numbers of test specimens are always preferable. If six test items are virtually identical in performance, then an $N = 6$ is acceptable (see Part II for the significance of N, the number of test specimens). If, however, there is an inherent variability in performance, 10% or greater, then a larger number of specimens should be tested ($N \geq 10$).

6. *Controls*: Research studies ideally are performed with controls against which the results of your studies on a new surgical procedure, a new dental material or a new pharmaceutical are compared. Controls provide an internal check on the validity of your test procedures and protocols.

a. A positive control is a test situation (such as a surgical procedure, established material or pharmaceutical product) that has a known, established, and accepted outcome. In evaluating the effectiveness of a new anti-inflammatory topical steroid, the experimental data might be compared with those found with the well-established practice of using hydrocortisone to treat the same condition. Likewise, the strength or solubility of a new dental cement might be compared to that for the traditional and time-honored zinc phosphate cement. Ideally, your test data will show an improvement compared to both the positive control as well as alternative approaches in procedure or material.

b. A negative control is a test situation in which no reaction should occur. In the evaluation of the corrosion resistance of implant metals, an example of the negative control might be immersion of a titanium implant in pure water, a situation in which no corrosion will occur. If a positive effect is found with a negative control, then one has to ascertain whether there might be an inherent fault in the test procedure or apparatus that causes something to happen when no reaction should occur.

Although a little reflection nearly always comes up with suitable negative and positive controls, it is not always possible. In the present cutting example, it is hard to conceive of a situation in which a dental bur will not cut anything (i.e., there is no negative control). A positive control can also be difficult since guaranteed cutting, for example, a high-speed handpiece and bur cutting through butter or dental cement, may not relate to the intended studies. In such cases, the control might be Bur A and all other burs are compared with the behavior of that bur under all the various test conditions.

7. *Data gathering and analysis*: Performing research involves both running of the experiment and recording the generated data.
   a. Hard copies (i.e., laboratory notebooks) of the data are excellent practice and it should always be borne in mind that the laboratory notebook is simply that and errors, misspelling, cross-outs, etc., should be left in place. Thus, the laboratory notebook is akin to patient notes with regard to making changes. The final report/dissertation/paper is the place for tidying things up, not the original data and its record. Data can be recorded directly on computer but this can lead to problems down the road, particularly if the hard drive fails.
   b. I personally prefer to analyze each set of data as it is generated. So, in the present cutting study, my approach would be to calculate the mean and standard deviation (see Statistics chapters) of cutting rates for say Type A burs at each cutting interval as well as, perhaps, the overall cutting rate over the specified number of cuts in the study. This initial analysis would also be performed for Type B, Type C, and all the other burs under that specific test condition. The process is repeated for each change in test condition, that is, different applied loads, coolant flow rates, chemomechanical effects, and so forth.

c. Continuous inspection and analysis of data has several advantages. Firstly, it provides the researcher with clearly identifiable milestones throughout the overall project. Secondly, it will indicate whether differences might exist between different burs or between cutting performances for different cutting conditions at an early stage. If large and/or unexpected differences are present, then one can recheck the test system, data gathering, or other parameter before too much time or effort has been expended. Finally, there is always a sense of accomplishment when one can point to a specific outcome at regular intervals.

d. Comparing one set of data with previously generated data, particularly if there has been a change in conditions, procedures, and testing personnel between the studies or even a long period of time between studies, can raise questions about the validity of such comparisons. Accordingly, one should always use controls to ensure that data from each series of tests are useful and complete in and of themselves. That way, artifacts and other unexpected results will be immediately apparent when the new set of data is inspected.

In this chapter, it has been assumed that the researcher is performing quantifiable studies that generate ordinal data. There are, however, other types of research that do not lend themselves to statistical analysis, for example, literature reviews, or parametric data analysis, for example, comparative studies based upon observations and scoring of clinical effects that are difficult to quantify. These topics are discussed in the next chapter. As noted above, statistical analysis will be addressed in Part II.

Non-Bench Research

To this point, the assumption has been that laboratory-based ("bench") research is to be performed and the discussion has been directed toward this objective. There are clear advantages to undertaking bench research (Table 6.1).

Clinically related and educational projects are often laboratory-based, at least initially. Microbiological studies, cellular experimentation, psychological tests, and so forth would be included in this category. Such studies are covered by standard protocols in their respective fields and since many projects are quantifiable and yield parametric data, they fall into the category of "bench" research. Many would-be researchers, however, do not have access to a laboratory or a multiplicity of test facilities. In such situations, perfectly viable alternative paths may be open to the prospective researcher, notably clinical research and literature reviews.

LITERATURE REVIEWS

Reviewing the literature is a necessary component of any research project, bench or clinical, and is required for research reports, theses, dissertations, and scientific papers; for simplicity, research reports, theses, dissertations, and scientific papers will be referred to as "reports." Literature reviews for reports are often restricted in length by the journal, university regulations, or by the intended application of the review. In other words, they must be focused and directed toward the subject matter of the report being written.

Literature reviews for reports are discussed in detail in Chapters 8 and 9 but some comments here might be useful. A comprehensive and critical review of the literature within a given field has merit in and of itself and most certainly "qualifies" as research. In fact, such reviews are extremely useful additions to the literature and are often quoted in research-based

Table 6.1   Advantages of bench research.

Precise null and alternative hypotheses
Accessible literature on previous/related studies
Definable and controllable test parameters
Available and reliable testing facilities
Reproducible test materials
Quantifiable test data
Parametric statistical analysis

scientific papers. The question is, how does one go about doing a "stand alone" literature review?

The Basics

1. *Interest in the subject*: The first rule in any writing should be interest. If you have no interest in the topic or, worse, even dislike it, it is very difficult to be motivated to write about that subject.
2. *Keep focused*: It is simpler, faster, and considerably easier to argue your case by going directly from discussion point A to discussion point B than to indulge in side trips or circumlocutions. The guideline for this direct line of argument is indicated in Figure 6.1. It is the preferred approach in most cases.

    When considering the line of your argument, although the pathway through items C, D, and E may be interesting, sidetracking directs attention away from the main thrust of your discussion. If, however, these subjects are really interesting, they can be introduced as subsections of the review you are working on provided you take care to emphasize what you are doing. This is most easily indicated by means of subheadings that make clear the relationship between the subsections and the main heading by numerical or alphabetical listings. This approach is indicated in Figure 6.2.

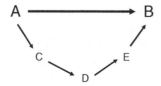

Figure 6.1   Direct is best.

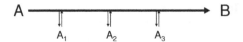

Figure 6.2 Incorporation of subsections into the review.

3. *Target the audience*: Having decided upon a topic to be reviewed, three questions have to be addressed regardless of the subject to be covered, namely:
   a. What is the purpose of the review?
   b. Is the nature of the review to be general (an overview of the subject) or specialized (directed at a limited area of a much larger field)?
   c. Where will it be published?
4. *Look at journals relevant to the topic area*: Journals relevant to the topic area should be carefully appraised, particularly their target readership and the style and level of the reviews they publish, before submitting a manuscript for publication. Many peer-reviewed journals in dentistry actively welcome review articles. There are also several continuing education (CE) journals (some of which offer honoraria to contributors) that rely upon reviews for their readership. Not all of these CE journals are peer-reviewed.
5. *Be aware of your readers*: It is essential that the review is pitched at the appropriate level for the intended readership. It is worth remembering that the same question can be asked in a freshman college examination and at a PhD *viva voce* but the depth of the response varies markedly with the situation.

   If your primary intended reader has specialized knowledge in the biological sciences, it is not a good idea to write a review with a large engineering or mathematics content. At best he or she will think you pretentious, at worst the reader might get an expert in that area to evaluate your work ... and that can be painful!
6. *Keep it simple* but not too simple: It is a reasonable assumption that your readers are experts in the field, otherwise they would not be reading your review. Accordingly, do not dwell on the basics since they should already know them although *briefly* touching on them can often be helpful to the reader. If you feel it is necessary to provide background material in greater depth, do so in an appendix. The decision on to what to omit or include should be based on common sense but when in doubt, seek advice.
7. *Keep it interesting*: Reading boring, colorless text is an interminable task. If you are bored writing the review, imagine what your reader is going through! You do not want to alienate the reader. The subject of writing style will be returned to in Chapter 9.

NON-BENCH CLINICAL RESEARCH

Clinical research can take many forms and pathways but predominantly involves patients and, as such, is fraught with difficulties because of the inherent variability within humans and animals. Common examples of clinical (non-bench) research include the observation and reporting of clinical signs and symptoms, modified and/or innovative surgical procedures, alternative treatment regimens, and the evaluation of pharmacological agents (new drugs). All of these research projects involve patients and, generally, large numbers of patients are necessary if statistically valid data are to be generated. Despite the difficulties, valuable research data can be mined by careful observation. It is noteworthy that Thomas Hodgkin, of the eponymous Hodgkin's Lymphoma, started his work on the disease based on observations of patients in an English village while still a very junior doctor in his early twenties.

Human studies require strict protocols, patient consent forms, and mandatory adherence to regulatory and ethical human study regulations. Animal studies are somewhat simpler in concept but are complicated by the difficulty of correlating and interpolating data from animal studies with humans. Further, the cost and availability of animal subjects, humane treatment requirements as well as antivivisection regulations are also important factors in animal studies.

Numerous factors bear upon clinical studies, and considerable bias can be introduced into research data if the myriad influences on human (and animal) responses to any treatment or device are not properly taken into account. Further, many factors are interrelated, or at least are influenced by each other.

It is impossible to cover all the factors that can impinge clinical research but some general comments might be useful with regard to research planning. Variations from the "norm," that is, an unexpected or atypical result or consequence of a treatment may due to gender, race, genetics, environment, or other effects. In an observational study involving the efficacy of a drug in patients across different cultures, for example, it is worth bearing in mind the relevant cultural variations that may impact on your field of study, such as the effect of dietary variations or the taking of health food supplements, which may contain ingredients that offset or neutralize the effects of drugs. A simple observational study of the efficacy or otherwise of a particular drug may therefore biased be due to an unaccounted-for variable. An example of dietary effects is that of vitamin B providing an alternative metabolic pathway for bacteria exposed to sulfonamide drugs and, consequently, neutralizing the drug's pharmacological efficacy.

In opinion-based research studies, the sample being evaluated must be truly representative of the population from which it is drawn. An example of socioeconomic effects on research is when the outcome of one twentieth-century U.S. Presidential election was "mis-called" because the pollsters conducted telephone interviews at a time when the majority of the population did not have telephones. As a result, the majority opinion was overlooked and the "favored" candidate actually lost the election because of biased poll-based advice.

It is impossible to identify, let alone negate or neutralize, all the factors and parameters that can impact, and distort, clinical studies. However, if the researcher is careful during research planning to identify and take into account factors that can affect the findings, then the research study will proceed far more smoothly. It must also be stressed that many effects suspected or proven to influence clinical outcomes have been identified in numerous studies and addressed in the literature.

It is always advisable to consult a biomedical statistician before embarking on any research study but it is particularly important with non-bench clinical studies due to the greater complexity of interpreting and analyzing results. In particular, researchers should gain detailed advice on the type and range of data to be collected and how it is to be evaluated, that is, the statistical analyses that will be performed, *before* starting the study. There is nothing more disappointing than to embark on an extensive project only to be told afterwards by a statistician that the cell sizes are too small for the effect under investigation to be meaningfully interpreted or that a confounding variable has not been adequately controlled.

RECORDING DATA FOR NON-BENCH RESEARCH

Many clinical studies make use of ordinal or parametric measurements (i.e., numeric data), for example, blood pressure, temperature, weight, blood chemistry, and other physiological parameters that are determined using a variety of instruments. These data are recorded and can be analyzed in a straightforward manner using parametric statistics. It becomes rather more difficult when comparative data are involved. Studies requiring evaluation of parameters such as the degree of inflammation, bacterial proliferation, and pain assessment all involve an individual's judgment and this can vary markedly depending upon the situation, patient response, and the assessing individual.

Research studies of this type can be handled in different ways, but commonly involve converting comparative data to ordinal values by means of scoring procedures. Pain, for example, can be assessed subjectively by the patient on a 10-point scale, ranging from unbearable (score of 10) to no pain (score of 0). The effectiveness of an analgesic is then rated by the patient as the change in pain score with administration of the new analgesic. In a multi-individual trial, it is possible to calculate the mean or average drop in pain scoring for the new analgesic compared with that for patients being treated with standard analgesics. The before-and-after pain scoring converts subjective assessments to ordinal values and data obtained from numerous patients can be statistically analyzed. Although pain scores, for example, are inherently subjective, this approach does permit an overall comparison of efficacy, with controls being the patients themselves. Obviously, placebos can also be administered (negative controls) as well as doses of analgesics of high known effectiveness being administered as the positive controls. The "placebo effect," however, is always a complication in such studies and may require more complex analysis. This is particularly true in the case of children where up to 30% of the response can be accounted for by a placebo effect.

Objectivity is hard to achieve in non-bench clinical research. One can have rating scales, for example, degree of impairment (mild, moderate, severe), but more commonly these would be on a rating scale such as 1–5 or 1–10 where only the direction would be indicated (i.e., 1 for mild and 10 for severe) without labeling the degrees in between. However, much more time has to be taken to evaluate interrater reliability because of the subjectivity of the measurements. If sufficient time is taken to clearly define what is being measured and to consider all the variables, which may confound the results, then extremely complex observational research becomes possible. An example would be the ratings of Ainsworth's strange situation that look at the separation reactions in young children. Good interrater reliability is achieved because the format is standardized and the ratings are measured via a video recording so that they can be compared more objectively. Children's reactions to a short separation can then be classified into a variety of categories (secure, insecure avoidant, insecure dismissive, or disorganized) according to carefully described behavioral criteria, which can be replicated by other researchers on the basis of the methods described.

Thus, in any non-bench clinical research, a rating scale must be established prior to the start of the study. Further, the examiners must be independent and, preferably, the subject to be measured should be calibrated using agreed and clearly defined standards so that comparable scores are achieved when multiple examiners evaluate the same situation. Rating scales typically might extend from 0 to 5 or 10 on an ordinal scale and all examiners should agree on the ratings. Using multiple examiners reduces the risk of bias in measurement (provided that the measurement itself does not have a systematic bias due to poor consideration of confounding variables). Multiple measurements allow statistical analysis of the before-and-after experiment conditions and the measured changes using the examiners' scores. However, the length of the scoring scale (i.e., the number of points) can influence the precision of the scoring system. More points on the scale should increase precision but the corollary is that a greater number of loci (score values) can introduce "shading" of the data. This effect is often to be seen on "reality" TV shows and competitive sporting events where a panel of judges rates performances on a multipoint scale. It is hard, for example, to really distinguish between the performance of an ice skater with a score of 9.1 and that of another competitor with a score of 9.2 or 9.3. It is also common in cases where longer ordinate or variable scales are used that raters tend to cluster their scores at certain points along the scale, for example, around the middle and ends of the scales, rather than spread ratings consistently along the scale.

Comparative data in which appraisals are based on opinions cannot be reduced to explicit or ordinal values; these are therefore difficult to analyze. Analysis may involve ranking the data or performing before-and-after comparisons but, as discussed under *Statistics*, techniques are available for this task, the approach being known as *nonparametric statistical analysis*.

On occasion, however, the results of clinical and some nonclinical studies simply cannot be quantified or subjected to statistical analysis. In such cases, not uncommon in many fields such as narrative data in psychiatry, psychology, and sociology, for example, the researcher must simply state the results in a summarized form and describe how conclusions were drawn from the presented data. For example, sociologists often collect large amounts of observational data, a classic example being Irving Goffman's study of an entire psychiatric system including the experiences of patients and staff at the National Institute of Mental Health in Washington, DC. Goffman went on to write a famous book of his study [Goffman, E. (1961) *Asylums: Essays on the Social Situation of Mental Patients and Other Inmates*. New York, NY: Doubleday]. Other examples include comparisons of scanning electron and optical microscopic histological images of materials or tissues in before-and-after treatment studies. In such situations, the reader can accept or reject the findings and their validity because all the requisite information such as micrographs is available for review.

CONCLUSIONS

Charles Prestwich Scott in the Manchester Guardian of May 6, 1926, wrote "Comment is free but facts are sacred." Both bench and clinical research findings have little meaning unless the data can be subjected to critical appraisal and analysis. The application of valid statistical analysis to research data is central to accurate and reproducible investigation. Without statistical analysis, opinion is simply that, an opinion that may or may not be substantiated. Although adverse and negative comments regarding statistics and statistical analysis are legion, they do permit the reader to assess the presented data and their interpretation because there is a logical basis for their explanation. This should be the aim of all research.

Nevertheless, opinion is very important when undertaking a literature review. With all due respect to Mr. Scott, the reviewer has a duty if not an obligation to present both sides of an issue, particularly if nonquantifiable data are under discussion. If anyone had listened to the unassuming dentist sitting in the audience when the Piltdown Man evidence was presented, the most famous paleontological hoax in history would have been still-born. Even though papers published in prestigious journals are subjected to peer review, hoaxes still make their way into such journals as *Nature* and *Science*. Merely because something has been published in a respected journal, it does not necessarily mean that the presented data and their interpretation are completely correct. Critical reviews should be just that, critical. The careful and critical reviewer actually is performing a service to science if he or she discusses both sides of an issue and attempts to indicate where scientific truth might lie. The review writer, however, must indicate where his or her opinion is being advanced, typically using a comment like "In the author's opinion ...."

Sources of Error and Avoiding the "Whoops" Factor

We all make mistakes, some of us more often than others, but we all make mistakes. These mistakes directly and indirectly affect our research and, more particularly, our research findings. While errors cannot always be prevented, it is possible to minimize them and their impact. Things change and so do people, and the effects wrought by these changes can cause chaos and confusion.

The following are basic guidelines on how to avoid preventable errors, many of them illustrated by anecdotes (in italics) of real experiences.

a. Balances, recorders, micrometers, and every other measuring device should be zeroed every day and certainly before each time measurements are made. All instruments should be calibrated using recognized standards at least once a week or more frequently depending upon use.

A new research student presented me some interesting data that were hard to explain. Careful questioning did not show anything was wrong until she was asked what the recorder chart speed had been. "Chart speed? What chart speed?" It came out that she had run one series of experiments at one chart speed and the second and third series at different speeds so the measurements were spread out differently, giving rise to the anomalous effects. Whoops!

The researcher had been given a course of instruction on the instruments she was using but enthusiasm overrode training and not all the test parameters were checked before each series of experiments was run.

b. Always, always, always run standards. It is hard to know if the unexpected is real or artifact when experiments have not been run with known standards at the same time and which can be used as comparators for the new data. The same rule applies to every reagent that is used.

When I was first employed at R&D in industry, I had been running an experiment that simply would not go the way it should have gone. After checking everything, it occurred to me to look at the chemicals I was using. The new container of potassium nitrate, supplied by a reputable manufacturer, in fact contained sodium sulfate. Whoops! Embarrassment all round and after the reagent was replaced, equilibrium was restored and things worked out the way they should have.

Although mislabeling of chemicals by manufacturers is rare, it does happen and when all else fails, it is worth checking the reagents that one is using.

c. Have replacements available, particularly for standard measuring instruments (e.g., pH and reference electrodes, chromatography columns, etc.). Comparing two or more instruments at the start of a study will eliminate a device that is not functioning properly, and avoid a lot of wasted time and disappointment.

Once I was called in to sort out why the retaining mesh for fiberglass filters was corroding when this problem had never been evident in previous years. Despite assurances that nothing had changed, it turned out that the company had switched to a different supplier of the fiberglass but they had not investigated the new material properly. It turned that the new material had a high content of hydrochloric acid and when the humidity changed, the acid was released and corrosion occurred. Whoops!

When the company went back to the old material, there were no more problems and saved literally hundreds of thousands of dollars per year. A clear example of what happens when necessary checks are not performed.

d. Measure twice, cut once! This adage of experienced carpenters is sound advice. It is often difficult and always a pain to have to go back and repeat something because an avoidable error in measurement was made early on.

A couple of years ago, I had two dental students working with me on the effect of soft drinks on extracted teeth. When I was proudly presented with a mass of data, it was immediately clear that something was very wrong and nothing seemed to add up. Careful questioning revealed that the students had not distinguished between dissolution effects on enamel and dentin and, worse, had not calculated the rates of attack on individual specimens. Instead everything had been lumped together. Whoops!

It was suggested to the students that there were marked differences in the compositions of enamel, dentin, and cementum and that this would significantly impact their dissolution in acidic beverages. Further, the students were politely introduced to the fact that individual specimens might vary in their behavior so that dissolution rates should be calculated for each specimen rather than en masse. Thereafter, the research went smoothly and useful data were generated.

e. What is said may not be what is heard! What might be clear and obvious to the speaker may be neither to the listener. Always check that the instructions you are giving are clear and precise as far as the listener is concerned. Conversely, what you hear may not be what was said.

A research student of mine was looking at dimensional changes of certain materials using a traveling microscope with a vernier scale. She made a series of measurements and got a set of data. I looked at the same specimens and got very different results but for no obvious reason. Eventually, it turned out that she took measurements from right to left while I measured from left to right. The rotatable vernier dial, however, had to be used for left-to-right measurements and gave incorrect values when used in the opposite direction unless corrections were made to the recorded numbers. Whoops!

It never hurts to watch how someone is measuring something—sometimes their approach is wrong or can give misleading data, other times their approach can be better than yours.

f. When all else fails, read the instructions. New versions of computer software, modified, improved or replacement instruments and, in fact, change of any sort can cause untoward problems. Even if one has been using a particular device or approach for years, it is always useful to check that what you are using or are accustomed to has not changed due to external factors.

While I was in industrial R&D with the Gas Council in the United Kingdom, I was running some electrochemical corrosion studies and periodically a strange effect occurred. What was odd was that the apparent artifact was reproducible only on certain days but not others. As it happened, my laboratory in Fulham, London, was next door to Fulham Gas Works and every so often the gas works released small quantities of sulfur oxides. These sulfur oxides got entrained in the test electrolytes and induced a secondary and very unexpected effect. Whoops!

Once I realized what was going on following careful checking of local pollution levels, the study was repeated using known levels of sulfur oxide additions and the effect was explained. Later, a paper based on these secondary studies was published.

g. Ask and ask again! In clinical studies, it is always worth checking, and rechecking, that the patient is not on any medications or is taking any of a variety of health supplements that can nullify or totally distort the effects you are investigating.

Patients often take vitamins that can provide alternative metabolic pathways for bacteria and thereby effectively neutralize the benefits of antibiotic therapy. This can occur with vitamin B and sulfonamides used for the treatment of certain conditions. Questioning patients on their diet and food supplements, for example, can avoid many treatment problems.

There was a classic case a few years back when a patient presented with acute aphthous ulceration of the oral mucosa, which responded to treatment. On subsequent recalls, however, the ulceration was sometimes present and absent on other occasions, regardless of any treatment provided, types of dental restorations and so forth. Then on one recall visit, the patient was observed to be chewing a particular brand of chewing gum which contained cinnamon flavoring. Inspection of the patient's medical history revealed hypersensitivity to cinnamon. Whoops! The condition was alleviated simply by changing the brand of chewing gum.

h. With computers and computer data processing, poor input data or errors in the programming for required calculations result in errors that may not always be apparent or readily detected. I have always performed one or two calculations by hand whenever I am using a computer to generate data from a mass of measurements. Dropping a decimal point, an incorrect line in the program and a host of other errors can easily arise with computers and their programming. Checking the data using a calculator and pen-and-paper calculations is a good safety net whenever one is analyzing data, and this has saved me from lots of but unfortunately not all errors.

An example of what can occur is when a computer or spreadsheet is programmed to convert measurements in feet and inches to meters and centimeters. If the conversion of 1 inch is taken to be 2.5 cm, 100 ft converts to 3000 cm (3 m). If the conversion of 1 inch is taken to be 2.54 cm, 100 ft converts to 3048 cm (3.048 m), an error of 1.6%, i.e., enough to cause problems.

Over a lifetime of research and research supervision, I have experienced countless examples of errors of omission and commission by others and, sadly, myself. Mistakes happen and none of us is perfect. However, following certain basic guidelines can avoid many problems and help one steer clear of the need to repeat studies. The importance of these guidelines should be immediately evident from the above anecdotes.

Reports, Theses, Dissertations, and Scientific Papers

At some time during their education or professional career, most people have to "write up" their work, be it an R&D report, a research paper, or a thesis/dissertation. Unfortunately, writing a coherent and comprehensible report, research paper, thesis, or dissertation (i.e., "report") is very challenging, particularly as most of us are unaccustomed to the task of writing.

The challenge is for you, the reader, to write a report on a research project. This generally implies work performed in the laboratory but also encompasses clinical research (medical, dental, or veterinary) and library-based work such as literature reviews. There is a further implication that the individual undertaking the research project did so with a particular end in view, for example, satisfying graduation requirements, a class assignment, a higher degree, or a scientific paper for publication. Whereas telling someone what to write or how to write is difficult, it is possible to offer guidance on a sensible approach to this task and provide advice on ways to simplify and speed up report writing.

The working assumption here is that the program of work has been completed, the data collected and statistically analyzed with appropriate conclusions drawn from the research findings. At this point, the hard work begins.

CONTENTS AND LAYOUT OF THE REPORT

All reports, regardless of their purpose (i.e., higher degree, internal company R&D report, or scientific paper), must adhere to a standard format although there may be differences in the details.

Reports are subdivided into sections, each section having a specific purpose and is designed to provide the reader with information that leads logically to the next section (Table 8.1).

Table 8.1 General format of reports.

Section	Content
Abstract	Overview and summary of the report
Introduction and literature review	The problem studied, previous work in the field and the basis for the study
Methods and materials	How the work was done
Results	What was found
Discussion	The significance of the findings
Conclusions	Relevance of the findings and what further work should be done

The designation of each section (and its specific content) can vary but the above is customary for virtually all reports. These sections will be discussed individually in the following chapters.

Dissertations and theses, depending on the university/college regulations, also may require such items as a title page, a contents page, often a brief *Curriculum Vita*, a summary of the literature review as well as the proposed program of work and the underlying research hypothesis. Some university regulations for theses and dissertations require a listing of tables and figures, as do many scientific journals. Some journals also require a brief biography ("bio") of the author(s).

Many scientific journals require that key or index words are provided with the manuscript. These are a collection of words that indicate the subject matter of your report. Placing these index words on the title page or on the same page as the abstract is useful as an indication of the content of the report and what the reader should be looking for in the text.

General guidelines

The following are general guidelines on the formatting of reports. Some of these will be returned to again in later chapters for emphasis but they are presented here for easier appraisal.

1. *Page numbering*: Every page of the report should be numbered consecutively. The position of the number can be a matter of choice or there may be specific guidelines that you have to follow. Some universities, for example, require the lead-in pages (title page, *Curriculum Vita* of the author, abstract, contents page, etc.) to have Roman numerals (i, ii, iii, …) and the body of the text to have Arabic numerals (1, 2, 3, …) but not all. Likewise, some journals have specific requirements for page numbering.

It should be noted, however, that if the page numbers are positioned at the bottom of the page, this can cause problems if footnotes are used for references or addenda to the text.

2. *New page for each section*: Although not mandatory, starting each section of a report on a new page aids clarity and provides a definite indication where one section is completed and a new one started.

3. *Line spacing*: The text should be double spaced for article submissions to journals and certainly makes all reports more readable.

4. *Abstract*: Abstracts for journal articles as well as submitted abstracts for scientific meetings often have definite word count limits. In such cases, use the "Statistics" facility under "Properties" in Word (or whatever word processor you are using) to check the word count.

5. *Justification*: Justified text improves the appearance of the text but some journals as well as university regulations may require nonjustified text. Check the requirements.

6. *Placement of tables and figures*: Articles submitted to journals usually have the tables and figures (and the references) placed at the end of the text. Placement of tables and figures in reports is often a matter of choice. Placing them within the body of the text may be useful if there is only a few of each and they are referred to only once. If, however, there are a large number of tables and figures and reference is made to them in different sections of the report, collecting them all together at the end of each section may be advisable. This arrangement makes it easier for the reader to review them and simplifies their inclusion since it is often a royal pain to insert figures and/or tables into text without messing up the arrangement of the text. This is particularly true if figures and tables have to be inserted in the text after it has been written and arranged.

If there are numerous figures, especially color diagrams and photographs, they will take up a lot of memory and the electronic files will be large. In some cases, the files can be so large that they are difficult to send by e-mail unless they have been converted to zip or PDF files. If the tables and figures are situated at the end of the text rather than scattered throughout, then they can be sent separately to the main body of the text.

7. *Font*: The selected font can markedly affect the readability of the text (Table 8.2). Font selection and the point size is up to you but one should always bear in mind that appearance can make a big difference in the acceptability of text, particularly if there is a lot to read. It is also worth remembering that if there is a space limitation, for example, an abstract submission has to fit within a certain size box, changing the font can maximize space utilization although any regulations/limitations

Table 8.2 Readability of different fonts.

Font	Appearance
Times New Roman 10 point	Is this readable to you?
Times New Roman 12 point	Is this readable to you?
Arial 10 point	Is this readable to you?
Arial 12 point	Is this readable to you?
Courier New 10 point	Is this readable to you?
Courier New 12 point	Is this readable to you?

on font size should be checked. Remember that if you change the font after the text is written, the pagination will change.

Use bold font and italics to emphasize certain aspects of the text (Figure 8.1) and often can change the meaning of the sentence. Overuse of boldface and italics, however, can be off-putting.

Although word processors make available a host of different fonts and font sizes, it is sensible to use the more common fonts, for example, Arial, Times Roman, or Courier, for the majority of applications. Whereas many of the available fonts are impressive and often artistic, their use can detract from the text.

8. *Check spelling*: Always use the spell check feature of your word processor to ensure that there are no glaring misspellings or strange instances of syntax in the text. Note that spelling errors are underscored in red on the monitor screen while syntactical problems are indicated by a green underscore. These markings are not apparent on printed copies.

It should be noted that word processors generally should not be relied upon for checking syntax since they cannot infer the meaning behind what

This is important.
This is important
This is important
This is important
This *is* important
This **is** important

Figure 8.1 Use of font changes for emphasis.

is being communicated. Consequently, it is sensible to read through everything on the monitor to look for errors that the word processor has spotted. Then, I suggest that the manuscript is printed out and read through again because corrections suggested by the word processor can often mangle the meaning of the text. These contextual changes may not be apparent on screen.

Further, a word may be used in the text that the word processor accepts because it is correctly spelled but its use is still incorrect. A simple example of this might be "The boys rode their bikes along the road." If this phrase had been written as "The boys road there bikes along the rode," the word processor might not pick it up the mistakes because of correct spelling except perhaps to suggest that *boys* should be written as *boy's* or *boys'*. Either alteration would still be wrong and mangle the sentence even more.

Introduction and Literature Review

The introduction and literature review is the second most important part of the report after the discussion. This section must provide a brief overview of the subject and indicate why the study was undertaken (Table 9.1).

WRITING THE INTRODUCTION AND LITERATURE REVIEW

The literature review, as the title suggests, requires the report writer to read and critically discuss previously published work (the literature) and the review must contain appropriate references or citations of that literature. It should be designed to center the reader's attention onto your particular problem by progressively narrowing the area of focus. In other words, you are using a funnel approach to restrict the amount of data reviewed in the report. This is shown schematically in Figure 9.1.

An essential point that cannot be overstressed is how the text is organized and written. I recently read a review of a new book and was struck by the opening comment: "As I flicked through this book I was initially disappointed by the long paragraphs. In some cases covering entire pages" (Ken Farrow in *Material World*, August 2008, p. 52). This issue will be discussed again in Chapter 15 under Notes on Writing.

The following should provide guidance on how to satisfy the requirements of an introduction and literature review.

1. *Introduce the subject*: Write an overall but brief review of the field of interest, and indicate where the research topic fits into this scheme.

Table 9.1 Objectives of the introduction and literature review.

Objective	Action
Set the scene	Provide a brief overview of the field of interest
Review general aspects	Provide general information that is relevant to the problem addressed in the report
Review specific aspects	Focus attention on the most important factors in the problem
Provide details	Review the literature that provides detailed information directly relating to the problem you are addressing in the report

2. *Define the problem*: Indicate the relevance of the research work and why the study was performed. Again, be brief—you are "setting the scene" for the literature review that follows.
3. *Provide a critical, logical, and coherent review of the literature*: Critically discuss previously published work. This review must be presented in a manner that helps the reader assess the research work within the report in the light of the available scientific information.
4. *Structure the literature review*: The larger the volume of available literature, the greater is the need for structuring the review. A well-structured review will also ensure that it progresses from the general to the specific smoothly and logically, as indicated in Figure 9.1.

Many approaches are possible but a very effective one is the "divide and rule" system. In this, the subject matter is divided, as far as possible, into subsections which are ordered so that the literature

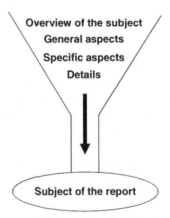

Figure 9.1 Schematic representation of the layout of a literature review.

review progresses logically. In other words, the funnel approach is used to relate the research problem to the general before presenting the particular. Each subsection should be discussed concisely.

This sectionalized approach requires careful consideration of the logical subdivisions but it will, in general, lead to a clearer presentation.

5. *Content of the literature review*: Deciding upon the content of the literature review is often difficult, and clearly varies with each research project and, indeed, with the interests and biases of the researcher. As an "opener," it is often useful to summarize the basic principles underlying the topic and if several views are current, then they should be presented at this point. Thereafter the most basic or general information should be discussed briefly in a separate subsection. In a clinical subject, this section would cover such factors as the patient general or oral health, diet, heredity, socioeconomic factors, etc., while in a biomaterials science project, the literature on the base materials would be reviewed. From this point, the publications covering clinical observations and/or treatments of a particular condition or the available information on a particular material or a class of materials would then be reviewed. An example of this structured approach is presented in Figure 9.2.

   Unless absolutely essential to the literature review, one should avoid quoting passages from the cited references. If such a passage is included, indicate that the text comes from someone else by means of quotation marks or italics while indenting clearly signifies that it is not part of the main body of text.

6. *Length of the literature review*: It should be noted that the introduction and literature review for an internal (Company) report or for a paper to be submitted to a scientific journal often differs from that of a thesis or dissertation. Internal R&D reports can be of any length but management may not look favorably upon exhaustive reviews of the literature. Scientific journals usually are limited on the space that can be devoted to a single communication and, generally, the introduction and literature survey for a research article will be limited to 2,000–3,000 words. While such restrictions are less common in dissertations, certain higher degree-awarding bodies do impose a maximum page limitation on the overall dissertation. Accordingly, brevity is always to be commended whatever the intended purpose of the report.

Finding the literature

Obviously in order to review the literature, one has to find it. In other words, what are the appropriate references to put into the literature review and how should one go about getting them? In today's internet and

THE REPAIR OF FRACTURED DENTURES

1. Introduction and literature review:

1.1 General introduction

Brief description of a denture, its design, fabrication, and its purpose

1.2 Denture design

Necessary design factors in complete dentures to ensure masticatory efficiency, retention, strength, and thermal stimulation of the underlying mucosa

1.3 Clinical considerations

1.3.1 Occlusal forces on dentures

1.3.2 Reaction of the denture to occlusal forces

1.3.3 Denture base movement in function

1.3.4 Deformation of the denture

1.3.5 Stress distribution in dentures

1.3.6 Long-term changes in dentures

1.4 Denture base materials

1.4.1 Desirable properties of denture bases

1.4.2 Physical properties of denture base resins

1.5 Prevalence and causes of denture fracture

1.6 The repair of fractured dentures

1.7 Summary of the literature review

1.8 Statement of the problem

1.9 Proposed program of work

Figure 9.2 Sample of the layout and organization of an introduction and literature review.

computer-driven world, things are considerably simpler and more convenient than in the past when everything relied upon diligent searching of current and past scientific journals. Nevertheless, it is still necessary to put some thought into this task and various sources can be searched for useful information.

The place to start is to look at recent papers in the field and check the references. If several papers cite the same publication or publications, then these are "must read" citations. For example, if several papers refer to a communication by Smith, Wesson, and Colt in say the journals *Nature* or *Science*, then you too should read this paper and include it in your literature review. Also, by looking at the published scientific literature over the past 2–3 years, you can get a good feel for what research is being performed in your specific area, indicate who is working in this area, and help identify other areas that impinge upon or are related to what you are doing. Reading recent papers also will help in deciding upon appropriate key words and/or authors for a computer search. Likewise, abstracts and presentations at scientific meetings are useful starting points.

International, and often large national, meetings function as a showcase for the latest research in the various specialties within a given field. The International Association for Dental Research (IADR), for example, attracts over 3,500 oral and poster presentations every year. The same holds true for virtually every specialty within medicine and dentistry. Many National and International Societies publish abstracts and/or proceedings of their annual meetings although there is a growing trend for these to be issued on CDs or memory discs/thumb drives. As a result, access is more difficult and may require membership of the organization or an efficient library system. Nevertheless, these compilations are excellent resources for identifying areas of research interest and the active workers within a given field. From there, it is relatively easy to identify and track down the recent and not-so-recent scientific literature.

Collected abstracts are very useful guides to relevant literature and will provide both titles and authors. Every field tends to have one or more such collections and reviewing them can save much time and effort. Many of these collected abstracts, for example, Index Medicus, Dental Abstracts, Oral Research Abstracts, Chemical Abstracts, Index to Dental Literature, and MEDLAR as well as the various Citation Indexes can be accessed online.

With regard to abstracts, a note of caution must be sounded. It is a natural temptation for people, when facing an extensive literature in a field, to simply rely only on abstracts for the literature review rather than read the entire paper. Abstracts, by their very nature, must be brief and they do not and cannot cover everything in the associated communication. Further, the information in the abstract is sometimes misleading and every so often downright wrong. It is not uncommon for the abstract to give a conclusion that cannot be justified by the evidence in the paper. Although relying solely on the abstract might appear to save time and effort, when a researcher does not bother to read the entire communication, he or she will miss out on a lot of solid and useful information. Usually when this happens, it can come back to haunt you.

Keyword-based computer search

In many respects, the internet is perhaps the best place to begin a major literature search but it does require some forethought.

1. First compile a list of key or index words or look up citations for a specific author or authors identified from the literature (as noted above).
2. Consult a librarian or information technology (IT) specialist and access the recommended database and start the search.

Despite sounding simple, some thought is necessary in order to maximize efficiency and effectiveness while avoiding wastage of countess hours when searching the internet. Entering only one or two terms in a Google or Yahoo search will yield tens of thousands of entries and it is an overwhelming task to even consider reviewing any but a relatively small number of "hits." Let us consider an example of what to do as well as what not to do:

An orthopedic surgeon proposes to evaluate a new type of bone cement recommended by a manufacturer for fixation of prosthetic hip joints and obviously he wants to access the literature in the field. An incautious person might use the following individual key words: bone, hip, cement, joint. Such a listing would provide the following number of "hits" and most of these would be useless:

Bone: 316 million covering composition, structure, morphology, physiology, strength and other properties of human, animal, fish, and avian bone

Hip: 801 million covering anatomy, biomechanics and physiology of human and animal hip joints as well as references to the fruit of the wild rose tree

Joint: 731 million covering the various articulations in human, animal, fish and avian anatomy, engineering structures, and even plumbing

Cement: 124 million covering Portland cement, masonry, dental adhesives, and resins

Clearly, one has to be specific regarding entries on the search topic line: "orthopedics" yields some 3,900,000 hits depending upon the search engine, "orthopedics and bone cement" results in 219,000 hits whereas "orthopedic bone cement strength" provides 86,900 hits. Modifying the information request with subcitations (e.g., compressive strength, solubility, adverse reactions) reduces the number of hits even further. Likewise, greater specificity, for example, "human hip joints," "orthopedic hip joint replacement," etc., will reduce the number of hits. When in doubt, consult with a librarian or IT specialist. These people are knowledgeable and, in my experience, are only too happy to help. It will save you hours of time and wasted effort by directing you to the most appropriate web sites.

The internet is an extremely useful resource in locating information within a field. While you might have to wade through dozens of web sites and numerous links even with good librarian or IT input, it is often possible to locate sources of information not readily available elsewhere and sometimes a completely different approach to the subject in question. Further, the internet/world wide web references may legitimately be cited in a report if they provide useful and directly relevant information. Some web sites actually provide citation guidance but an example of how to do this would be:

National Institutes of Health Consensus Development Conference Statement (1983). Dental Sealants in the Prevention of Tooth Decay. NIH Consensus Statement Online 1983 Dec 5–7;4(11):1–18. Available at: "http://text.nlm.nih.gov/nih/cdc/www/40txt.html." Accessed April 1, 2000.

However, the information that comes from a computer search is determined by a number of factors and rarely can be considered to be definitive. Not every published scientific paper gets into the computer database and while many databases will duplicate information, each will have different selection criteria for what is included. Poor selection of key words by an author can result in that paper being excluded from a database because the selected key words did not fit the criteria. Also, each time a search is performed, different information may come up even with the same key words, especially when different databases are used. Finally, the information (references) in a database will only be as good as the information included in that database. Many older publications (and numerous newer references) are missed because the computer search did not pick them up or they simply were not present in the database.

A useful feature of many databases is the "related articles" feature. Reviewing such references sometimes may take you down the wrong path but as often as not, these related articles can provide unexpected information relevant to your topic.

References

There are different approaches to the inclusion (citing) of references, and the one used can be a matter of choice but may also be dictated by the intended target of the report.

a. *Footnotes or endnotes*? Most scientific journals and reports place the references as endnotes. When the bibliography of cited references is placed at the end of the text (i.e., endnotes), it is easier for the reader to switch from the body of the text to the bibliography and back when going through the report. Also, most word processors have an endnote feature and there also are available proprietary software that are even more efficient and versatile [see (c) below].

b. *Calling up references (literature citations)*: For an internal report or a thesis/dissertation, literature citations may often be a matter of personal choice. Many journals and graduate schools, however, are very specific on how references are called up in the text and, indeed, how they are compiled in the bibliography. Always check with the author's instructions for any journal before submitting the manuscript and, preferably, before writing it.

c. *References: by author name and publication year or by number*? There are pros and cons to both approaches to referencing the literature.

   If the references are cited in the format of author name and year in the text, then changing a reference or adding additional references is a simple matter. Further, if there are several citations of the same reference within the text, the writer does not need to keep track of numbering of the references to avoid duplication. The disadvantages are that the writer has to decide whether the references in the bibliography are listed in alphabetical order or chronologically. This is generally not a problem with a bibliography containing relatively few references but it can be a headache when a large number of references are cited. Further, most word processors with built-in endnote (reference) capabilities insert numbers or letters in the text when citing the literature rather than citations to authors and publication year. In other words, literature references with common word processors are in the form of *Jones, Smith and Harbuckle*[2] rather than *Jones, Smith and Harbuckle, 1998*. More sophisticated word processors and specialized reference software often have greater capabilities in this regard. Such software will often automatically format references in accordance with the requirements of specific journals.

   A further consideration is that the citing of a large number of references by author name and year within the text makes it rather difficult to read. Compare the following two presentations of the same information:

A. Determining the crystal structure of antigens is thought to be central to understanding their function [Robinson, 1997; Jones, 1998; Cartwright, 1998; Smithson, 1999; Venables, 1999]. The techniques used for elucidating antigen crystal morphology include x-ray crystallography [Richards, 1996; Venables, 1999; Storey, 1999], Raman spectroscopy [Robinson, 1997; Cartwright, 1998; Peters, 1999], multidimensional NMR [Plodger, 1998; Smithson, 1999; Reynolds, 1999], etc.

B. Determining the crystal structure of antigens is thought to be central to understanding their function.[1-5] The techniques used for elucidating antigen crystal morphology include x-ray crystallography,[5-7] Raman spectroscopy,[1,3,8] multidimensional NMR,[4,9,10] etc.

Citing references by number, as in approach B, makes the text easier to follow but it does require the writer to pay careful attention to the numbering of the references. This can be a problem when there are multiple citations of one or more references. If a particular publication has been cited at different places within the text and references are cited by number, each citation of that particular reference should NOT be given a new number. Instead, only use the original or first number for that citation regardless of how many times it is cited or where it is cited in the text.

To make life as easy as possible with the literature review, I adopt the practice of writing short summaries (two or three sentences) of what has been read and the salient points that need to be covered and always make a note of the author name(s), journal name, and publication details. My personal preference is to number the various summaries and place them in a separate file from which they can be pulled out as and when needed. In the case of a literature review for a scientific paper or even a book, I find it is most convenient to put the references in parentheses as author name and year throughout the text and keep a separate note of each and every reference. Finding this information at a later stage can be a real "bear" so I like to keep track of things while writing.

After notes have been made on everything, they are then organized as indicated above using a cut-and-paste approach. After the summaries are placed in order within separate sections, it is also useful to write at the end of each section a brief summary of the information contained in that section. Following this approach, writing the literature review is then reduced to tidying up the notes and ensuring that the review is organized in a logical order. Writing the summary simply involves melding the separate section summaries into one.

Finally, when I am satisfied with what I have written and that it all hangs together, the format of reference citations is changed to that required by the specific journal to which I intend to submit the paper. Using this approach, keeping track of the references is automatic because I have kept a list and there is a considerably reduced risk of duplicating or misplacing references.

Summary and program of work

The introduction and literature review should be concluded with a brief statement of the problem that you have investigated, why you performed the study and the approach that was used.

In the case of a dissertation/thesis, the literature review should be followed by a 1–2 page summary of the information that you have reviewed in detail. The summary should focus attention on what you consider to be the most important facets of the literature on the subject. This should be followed by a statement of the problem, that is, a statement of what you want to do and why you are doing it based on the available information in the literature. Where appropriate, the underlying scientific hypotheses should be stated here. Finally, there should be a proposed program of work, namely a brief outline of your intended research project.

Methods and Materials (Experimental)

This section of the report presents the experimental methods and the materials (be they chemical, metallurgical, human, or animal) used in the investigation. Brevity and clarity are essential. If a particular instrument has been used, state what it is and specify the model number and give the manufacturer and address in parentheses, for example, a Model 8937 gas chromatograph (Allied Analytical Instruments, Bethesda, MD). It is unnecessary to give also the supplier's name, the cost, the year of manufacture or similar data unless it is strictly relevant to the study. It is also a valuable maxim that one picture is worth a thousand words, and a clearly labeled diagram usually is worth two thousand.

Unless perfectly standardized and well-established procedures (or the instrument and/or product manufacturer's instructions) have been followed, the experimental method should be given. Such details are necessary to:

a. Clearly indicate what your experimental work entailed
b. Help account for and explain any differences between your findings and those of others
c. Allow the study to be repeated by others if necessary

The precision or accuracy of measurement should also be stated clearly, for example, dimensions were measured with XYZ micrometer to ± 0.01 mm and specimen weights were determined to ± 0.0001 g using an $ABCD$ balance.

Pertinent information should be given on the materials or subjects/patients used in the research work, noting the fact that any research involving human or animal subjects requires institutional review board approval:

1. *For human patients*: Indicate sex, general and/or oral health, family history, age (and race if pertinent).
2. *For animals*: Indicate sex, physical condition, history, age and living conditions.
3. *For materials*: Provide details of composition, manufacturer, batch number, date of manufacture, purity, pretreatments, etc.

It is often useful to provide a table of the test materials when several different products have been tested. The table should provide details of the trade and generic names, type of material, manufacturer and location of manufacturer, batch number, and date of manufacture. This approach simplifies writing of the text since one can then simply state: *"The materials used in the study are summarized in Table xxxx."*

Similarly, one can summarize the experimental or test regimens in a table, which is very useful when several different groups of specimens were tested. This sort of table also serves as a useful guide to the different test procedures that the reader can refer to when reviewing the results of the study.

Finally, the statistical analysis techniques used and the predetermined significance level should be stated. Typically, for parametric (or number-based) data, a one-way or two-way ANOVA (analysis of variance) is performed to determine whether differences exist in the data. Thereafter, a multicomparison test such as a Scheffé or Tukey HSD test is performed to identify where the differences lie at a predetermined significance level, for example, $\alpha = 0.05$, 0.01, or 0.001. A similar approach should be used for nonparametric (comparative) statistical analyses of data. Statistical analysis is covered in Part II.

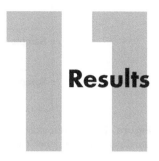

Results

This section of the report presents the findings or results of the research study, but only the results at this juncture. A logical presentation should again be attempted and it is preferable to present the results of a multi-faceted project in separate subsections. Wherever possible, tabulated or graphical data should be presented although the data should be summarized in the text. The tabulated data should include mean values and their standard deviations, for example, 15.5 ± 2.31 g/mL, where the first number (15.5) is the mean value and the second number (2.31) is the standard deviation. It is also useful to place the coefficient of variation in parenthesis beneath the data in the table. When data are presented this way, the table should have a footnote identifying the components of the data, as shown in Figure 11.1.

It should be noted that if the data are measured to a precision of ± 0.1 mm, the data should not be quoted to more than one decimal place. This is an important consideration since computer software spreadsheets will perform calculations and show the results to 5 or 6 decimal places. If measurements were made to a maximum of 1 decimal place, for example, dimensions to ± 0.1 mm, presenting data to 0.00001 mm is both illogical and wrong.

The statistical analyses should be presented in this section and the data can be tabulated with a brief commentary in the text. The table in Figure 11.2 shows an example of data comparisons with the significance levels identified beneath the table.

If the research involved a number of different studies, particularly if the studies were independent of each other, it is useful to put the results of each separate study in a subsection. This aids clarity and allows one to discuss the findings of each substudy separately before combining all the data in the final summary of the discussion.

It is worth repeating here that, despite the temptation to do otherwise, only the findings or results of the research study should be presented in

	Method A	Method B
Sample 1	15.5 ±2.31* (14.9%)	14.9 ±1.9 (12.8%)
Sample 2	17.3 ±3.1 (17.9%)	15.6 ±4.7 (30.1%)

Figure 11.1 Presentation of research data in tabular form [where *: mean value ± standard deviation (coefficient of variation, %)].

this section. Placing all the results tables and diagrams together at the end of the section will help the reader evaluate the data *en masse* as well as help you to review everything when writing the discussion.

PRESENTING THE DATA

While presenting the research findings in both tabular and graphical form is generally acceptable for theses and in R&D reports, it may not be acceptable in journals due to space (and often cost) limitations. Nevertheless, the presentation of data in graphical form does clearly demonstrate similarities and differences within the data. This is shown in Figure 11.3 for the data in Table 11.1 plotted using an Excel spreadsheet.

Looking at the data in Table 11.1 and Figure 11.3, it is apparent that there may be differences between samples A.1 and A.2 for Method A and samples B.1 and B.2 for Method B. Further, the scatter in the data for Method B, indicated by tie bars, appears to be greater than that in Method A.

If, however, the coefficients of variation for the data are tabulated (Table 11.2), the scatter in the two sets of data is more apparent.

The data for samples A.1 and A.2, and those for B.1 and B.2, appear to be very similar but there may be differences in the data sets for the two test methodologies. If the A.1 and A.2 specimens were basically the same

	Sample A	Sample B	Sample C
Sample A	—	ns	s
Sample B	ns	—	s
Sample C	s	s	—

Figure 11.2 Tabulation of statistical analyses. ns, non-significant ($P > 0.05$); s, significant ($P < 0.05$).

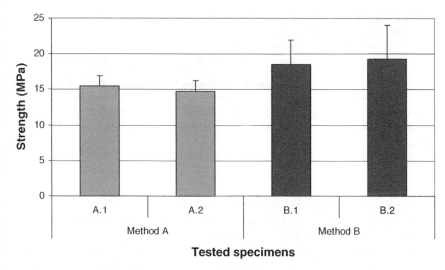

Figure 11.3 Graphical presentation of the data in Table 11.1.

material and likewise if B.1 and B.2 were different batches of the same product, then one might expect comparable data for samples A.1 and A.2, and for the B.1 and B.2 samples. Statistical analysis does in fact show no significant difference between A.1 and A.2 or between B.1 and B.2. There are, however, significant differences between A.1 and B.1 and between A.2 and B.2, indicating that the two test methods yield different findings with ostensibly the same materials.

Integrated software such as Microsoft Word and Microsoft Excel allows easy insertion of data from spreadsheets (and Microsoft Power Point) directly into text documents. The graphics capabilities of these programs permit a number of different ways of presenting data to be undertaken relatively easily. Similar capabilities exist in other bundled software packages such as those provided by Corel for PC use and the iWork package (pages, numbers, and keynote) for the Mac.

Table 11.1 Strength data (in MPa) for two test methods A and B and two series of specimens tested using each method.

	Method A		Method B	
	Series 1	Series 2	Series 1	Series 2
Mean value ± standard deviation	15.5 ± 1.4	14.7 ± 1.5	18.5 ± 3.5	19.3 ± 4.7

Table 11.2 Strength data (in MPa) for two test methods A and B and two series of specimens tested using each method.

	Method A		Method B	
	Series 1	Series 2	Series 1	Series 2
Mean value ± standard deviation (coefficient of variation, %)	15.5 ± 1.4 (9.03)	14.7 ± 1.5 (10.20)	18.5 ± 3.5 (18.92)	19.3 ± 4.7 (24.35)

The above findings and those obtained from statistical analysis would be presented in the results section of the report. There should, however, be no discussion other than a statement of the findings. It should also be noted that tables and figures should be clearly labeled so that the reader can see instantly what these items show without having to dig through the text for explanations.

A word of caution should be introduced regarding presentation of data. When data are plotted using Excel or PowerPoint, it is essential that you tell the computer what you want to plot. The data in Table 11.3 can be plotted in different ways (Figures 11.4 and 11.5).

The line plot (Figure 11.4) simply presents the data and suggests a sudden rise in the measured parameter after 8 days. If the data are plotted using an x–y or scatter diagram (Figure 11.5), a different picture of the data emerges.

Only the scatter diagram (x–y plot) (Figure 11.5) truly indicates the relationship within the data. In particular, the linear correlation between the measured parameter and time is immediately apparent.

Table 11.3 Data measurements over 20 days.

Time (days)	Series A
1	2
3	5
4	8
7	11.5
8	14
17	25
20	32

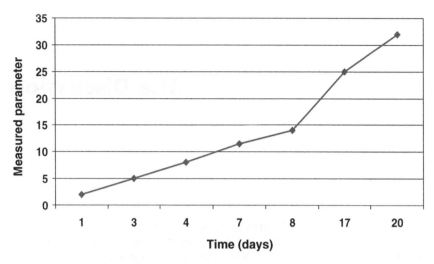

Figure 11.4 Line plot of data in Table 11.3.

Incorrect and/or incautious plotting of data is relatively common. Not only does it inhibit proper interpretation of the data but will cause readers of the report to question whether other mistakes have been made. This can be disastrous in the case of higher degree dissertations and for papers submitted to scientific journals.

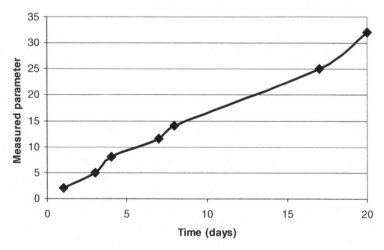

Figure 11.5 *x–y* (scatter) plot of data in Table 11.3.

12

The Discussion

The discussion is the most important section of a report. In this section, the author interprets the findings and discusses their significance. The discussion is also the section in which the data from your study are compared and contrasted with the findings of other workers. The discussion also serves as the forum for new theories or explanations of existing data from other studies.

DATA ANALYSIS

Correlation of all the results, particularly those presented in separate subsections, should be performed in this section. In particular, the author needs to indicate where the findings from different aspects of the overall study support each other and lead to the same conclusion. However, if differences exist among the findings in different parts of the same study, they must be accounted for in this section. Likewise, differences between the results of the present study and those presented in the literature must also be explained.

It should be noted, for example, that the observed differences can arise from a variety of sources, including the testing methodology, sampling technique or as a result of batch variations in the experimental materials. But, regardless of the source, such discrepancies must be accounted for or at least rationalized by valid argument. This can be particularly true when statistical analysis shows no significant difference in two sets of data while simple (visual) comparison of the mean values suggests that large differences exist. An example is the following set of data. Table 12.1 shows the mean values for four sets of data and inspection suggests an obvious difference between Group D and Groups A and B, and possibly Group C also. Differences in the scatter of the four data sets are shown in Figure 12.1, a plot of mean values with standard deviations indicated as

Table 12.1 Mean values (and their standard deviations) of four data sets.

Test group	Mean value
A	25 ± 1.2
B	22 ± 2.1
C	19 ± 2.3
D	17 ± 12.2

tie bars. For convenience, the discussion will be confined to Groups A and D, the two groups with the highest apparent difference.

Statistical analysis of the data, however, indicated no significant difference between Groups A and D. This seemingly nonsensical difference between what might be intuitively obvious and what was found is a dilemma that researchers often face.

Inspection of the data clearly indicates that the scatter for Group A, with a coefficient of variation of 4.8%, is markedly less than that of Group D, which has a coefficient of variation of 71.8%. Clearly, the scatter in the two sets of data causes the unlikely absence of difference in the two sets of data. In fact, it is not so much the scatter within the data in and of itself that causes the problem, but the number of specimens in each test group. It is a "quirk" of statistical analysis that comparisons of data sets that have a high degree of scatter (i.e., large standard deviations and coefficients of

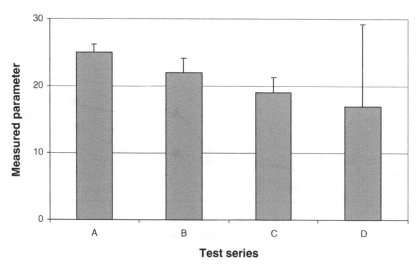

Figure 12.1 Plot of mean values of data sets (standard deviations presented as tie bars).

variation) require large numbers of specimens (i.e., a large N) for statistical significance to be demonstrated. In the present example, no significant difference ($P > 0.05$) was found when $N = 12$ for each group but there was a significant ($P < 0.05$) difference when $N = 20$ for both groups. Therefore, the apparent anomaly in the statistical analysis was due to a small sample size. In such a case, the researcher would conclude that the use of larger sample sizes would ensure that apparent differences might become real (i.e., statistically significant) differences. Nevertheless, the researcher still has to account for the fact that there are differences, particularly in the amount of scatter, between Groups A and D.

The above problem is actually quite common in research. On many occasions when I have reviewed/refereed manuscript submissions for scientific journals, I have had to draw the attention of authors to such apparent anomalies and suggest that they address the issue in the discussion section of the paper.

RESULTS VERSUS DISCUSSION

A question that often arises during report writing is "What goes where?" In most cases, there is a clear distinction between what should go into results and what more properly should be in the discussion. Sometimes, however, there is a degree of overlap and then decisions have to be made. An example of this might be the data plotted in Figure 12.2. In this

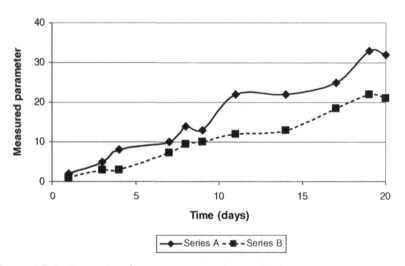

Figure 12.2 Two series of measurements made over 20 days.

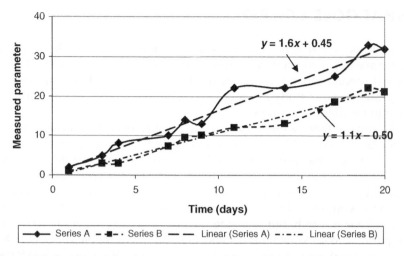

Figure 12.3 Plotting data from Figure 12.2 with trend lines and their equations.

example, two series of hypothetical measurements were made over a 20-day period and both curves appear to have a linear relationship between the measured parameter and time. These data correctly should be presented in the results section.

When one wishes to analyze the data further, problems arise. Plotting trend lines and deriving the corresponding equations (Figure 12.3) now may enter the realm of discussion.

The trend lines clearly indicate linearity in the data and the differences in the two equations ($y = 1.6x + 0.45$ and $y = 1.1x - 0.5$) suggest that while the two series are similar, they may not be identical. Statistical analysis will indicate whether these differences are significant and the presence, or the absence, of a difference requires discussion. Since the trend lines, their equations, and the use of statistical analysis to determine the significance of any difference between the curves are an extension of the basic results, these figures and their analysis should be in the results section. Appraisal and explanation of the findings, however, clearly belongs to the discussion section.

As an aside, it should be noted that the curves and their trend lines are readily plotted in Microsoft Excel (see Part II).

The rationale adopted in the above example should be adopted in all cases where there might be a problem deciding where to place data and their extensions, notably calculations and replotting of the data. Clearly there are always exceptions but unless there is a major change or shift in the way the data are treated or analyzed, that data should always be placed in the results section.

WHAT GOES WHERE?

It is a basic rule that no references should be placed in the discussion if they have not been cited in the introduction and literature review. This is a good precept when writing the discussion, particularly when the data generated in your study are compared with the findings of other studies cited in the literature survey.

As always, there seldom are hard-and-fast rules and, on occasions, exceptions are acceptable and/or necessary. If, for example, a new mechanism or theory has been developed that impinges on your data, it is acceptable to refer to this in the discussion and, obviously, cite the reference even though it was not raised in the introduction and literature review. Likewise, you might find some published work that does not directly relate to your research, but "outside the box" thinking suggests that there are parallels with your findings and those in a different and possibly totally unrelated field. Again, citing this work in the discussion when it has not been addressed previously is acceptable.

There are other instances when "breaking the rule" is acceptable. It is not uncommon to find that the measuring system you are using can introduce aberrations in the data or you have come across a new or better way to interpret your data. Modifications in technique or interpretation might not directly influence the rationale behind your study as outlined in the introduction and literature review but they may impact the discussion. Again, they should be cited in this section even if they were not addressed previously.

NOTES ON WRITING THE DISCUSSION

1. The number one rule with a discussion is that it should not restate the results unless it is absolutely necessary for the main thrust of your argument.
2. Do not forget the basics! There are legions of reports that have been wrecked because the researcher forgot the basics and overlooked the fact that the findings were perfectly obvious when viewed in the light of established theory.
3. Ideally, in the discussion, the findings of your study are discussed and compared and contrasted with the findings of other studies. In order to do so, you might have to briefly review the underlying theories and science of your study before you embark upon the discussion.

   While it might be acceptable and sometimes necessary, devoting a lot of space to restating basic principles may be questionable unless those principles are unique, difficult to locate in the literature or are absolutely essential to the thrust of your argument. Although rare, it is possible that your findings demolish established theory and, therefore, it might be useful to review the traditional view before espousing your new theory or mechanism. In such cases, citing those basic principles in the discussion rather than in the literature review might be another exception to the rule mentioned above.

4. Although it may be obvious, it is always a good idea to review your data and make short notes on what you have found before starting to write the discussion.

5. Likewise, an evaluation of the introduction and literature review is useful in focusing the mind on what you have done in relation to what other work is out there. It is astonishing how often one misses the significance of something even when you wrote the review.

6. Although discussed previously, as it will be again in later chapters, it is worth restating the axiom that paragraphs should be kept short. Each facet of your data should be reviewed and discussed separately, preferably in a new paragraph each time.

7. If the results have been presented in subsections, then each subsection can be discussed in turn. However, the significance and interrelationship of all these separate and often disparate discussions must be brought together within the discussion, usually toward the end.

8. Do not draw conclusions unless necessary since that is the designated role of the conclusions section.

9. Bad science will always be bad science no matter how elegantly it has been written up. Inadequate discussion of the data or glossing over inconvenient findings is bad science.

10. Always remember that a negative finding is a positive result. Plans go awry in everything, including research but explaining why something did not happen can be as big if not a bigger challenge than accounting for an expected positive finding or outcome.

11. Indicate any major advances in theory or practice that have come out of your research.

12. Where possible, compare the advantages and disadvantages of your approach to that of others working in the same field.

13. Indicate any limitations in the study and, hopefully, provide recommendations for addressing these issues.

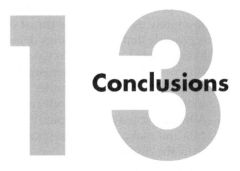

Conclusions

The first thing that many readers of reports (and reviewers of manuscripts) read after the abstract is the conclusions. While this might seem like reading the last couple of pages of a detective novel, and possibly spoiling the surprise, it does serve the useful purpose of "clueing the reader in" to what he should look for when reading the complete report. As a result, the conclusions have almost a disproportionately large importance.

The conclusions section of a report serves several purposes, namely to:

1. Review, summarize, and draw conclusions from the discussion
2. Indicate the significance of the findings
3. Provide recommendations for further work
4. Indicate, in the case of biomedical research, the clinical significance and applications of the research. The significance and applications of the research obviously also apply for nonbiomedical research work

The conclusions should summarize in a logical manner the preceding discussion. Any new theories or reaction mechanisms that have been propounded should be reiterated. The clinical significance of a purely scientific biomedical investigation should always be given while for a clinical investigation, recommendations for alterations in practice or procedures need to be stated.

Finally, there should be a brief summary of the overall project. That is, a clear statement of the work performed, what was achieved, the importance of the findings, and what further research work can be performed. The latter is quite important, if only to acknowledge the fact that no study, however comprehensive, answers every question that can and should be raised about the topic in question. Also, the recommendations for further work will suggest to the up-and-coming researcher, or the would-be researcher looking for a project, what areas he or she might wish to focus on in the field. Such recommendations also have the merit of establishing a quasi-claim to being the first within a field of study.

The same rules on good and effective writing apply here as in other sections of the report. Although there appear to be no strict guidelines, it is not uncommon for authors to present their conclusions and recommendations for further study as a series of bullet statements, particularly if there is several of each. Others tend to follow the more traditional narrative approach of continuous text. How the information is communicated in a report is probably a matter of choice but with poster and PowerPoint oral presentations, the bullet approach is a definite "must."

14

The Abstract

The abstract provides an overview and summary of what the report contains, and it should be brief but must also be accurate. In fact, the one certain item of information, other than the title and author, that will be turned up in a literature search is the abstract, particularly with the internet searches. Accordingly, the abstract allows the potential reader of a journal article, for example, to decide whether to read the article immediately, "back-burner" it or to ignore the article completely if it is outside an area of interest. In effect, the abstract has the same function as a movie trailer, drawing the reader into the manuscript and providing an indication of the contents. A poorly written abstract will deter readers while inaccuracies in an abstract can be repeated forever, particularly with individuals who rely on abstracts rather than the entire paper for their information.

Given this important role, the abstract should be written in such a way that it identifies the key issues within the report. It should not simply be a reiteration, albeit in condensed form, of what the report is about. In many cases, the abstract is required to be structured and this is discussed below.

ABSTRACT FORM AND CONTENT

The format of a structured abstract should adhere to the following general outline or basic format:

Purpose: A brief overview of why the study was undertaken.
Materials and methods: What you did and how you did it together with a
   brief description of any statistical tests.
Results: A brief statement of what you found. If you produced numerical
   data, give mean values and their standard deviations and summarize
   the results of statistical analyses. State the main finding in a single sentence.

Conclusions: Concisely indicate the significance of your principal find-
ing(s).

Whereas the basic format for a structured abstract is similar, different journals may require specific formats and, indeed, some journals may prefer a
less ordered abstract.

ABSTRACT LENGTH AND CONTENT

The length of an abstract will vary with the intended audience, that is,
whether it is for a professional or scientific journal, an internal (company)
report, or a dissertation. Typically for a published paper in a journal, the
abstract comprises 400–700 words (or 1–2 pages of typescript) but the
length will vary with the nature of the submitted manuscript and the journal. A word count of 700 or so words is typical for abstracts submitted to
national and international meetings.

A clinical report to be published in a journal, for example, will generally have an abstract that concisely describes the content of the report and
the benefits to the patient and/or clinician from reading it. Likewise, the
abstract of a scientific (nonclinical) paper will summarize the purpose of
the study, methods and materials used, the findings of the study and indicate, briefly, the discussion and the conclusions drawn from the results.
Since some journals encourage very long abstracts, it is worth inspecting
recent issues of the journal you intend to submit to in order to see what
that journal favors in the way of an abstract. It is also worth checking on
what the format of the abstract should be since formats can vary with different journals.

Abstracts for internal (company) reports tend to be longer in length
than those for submission to professional and scientific journals. In particular, the abstract of a research report serves the same function as the executive summary of financial and marketing reports. The busy executive will
scan the abstract before deciding whether or not to read the report and,
therefore, the abstract for this purpose tends to be focused on the results,
discussion, and, particularly, the conclusions of the report. The "hows"
and "whys" of a project within an internal report tend to be less important than for journals since management generally have a very good idea
of why (and often how) the study was performed. A poorly written abstract will deter management from reading the report and this can reflect
badly on the writer.

A dissertation or thesis also will generally have a much longer abstract
than a published paper. The summary of the literature review should be
condensed down to one or two paragraphs, in effect, a condensate of the

summary of the literature review. Methods and materials should be brief and indicate, in broad terms, what was done, with what and how. The results component should be longer but again must be concise and to the point. Likewise, the discussion and conclusions components should be brief and encompass only the most important findings and their significance. A concluding paragraph stressing the most important finding and its impact on the field of interest sets the reader up for what is to follow in the report.

KEY WORDS

Many scientific journals require that key or index words be provided with the manuscript. These are a collection of words that indicate the subject matter of your report. Placing these index words on the title page or on the same page as the abstract is useful as an indication of the content of the report and what the reader should be looking for in the text. These key words are also the indicators used for the inclusion of papers in data bases. Poor or inappropriate key word selections will limit the readership of your work because they may not be able to find it in a literature search.

It should be noted that requirements for key words can vary with the journal and, in some cases, the key words should not repeat words or terms used in the manuscript title.

WHEN TO WRITE THE ABSTRACT?

At what point in the report writing should one write the abstract? This is a matter of choice. I often write the abstract after I have written the bulk of the text so that I am completely familiar with the report content and can highlight the important features. Others may write the abstract first so that they can organize the text better as they write; that is, the abstract provides a road map to the body of the report. It really does not matter which approach you adopt as long you remain focused and ensure that the abstract is accurate and does justice to the report.

A problem that can arise if the abstract is written before the report is what might politely be called obfuscation. When an abstract is written quasi-independently of the report, there is often a tendency to write what one hopes was found rather than what was actually demonstrated. This may not be that uncommon a problem given how often the abstract of a paper appears to bear little relation to what was reported in the paper. All report writers are strongly discouraged from adopting this practice.

Writing Style and Technique

This far, attention has focused on the basic format of the scientific report and little has been said on how to write. Regardless of one's experience and indeed the subject matter of a report, it is always a difficult task to undertake writing anything, even a letter. There are, however, a number of things that one can do to assist in this task.

Before starting to write, sit back and read through all your notes so that everything is fresh in your mind. Then you can start. However, it is virtually impossible to define the rules of writing because no such rules exist and even if they did, they would probably be largely ignored by most people. Accordingly, the following suggestions are offered as a guide to be followed rather than rigid "rules of writing."

- Keep the average sentence length to 30 words or so. The optimum length of a sentence is 3 lines or less, that is, 24–27 words. Long sentences are unwieldy and extremely long sentences, viz., 5 lines or more, are indigestible. Never write sentences so long that they form a paragraph of their own.
- Write simply, clearly, and use ordinary (common or garden) English expressions.
- Keep it simple. It is better to say "round holes" than "circular orifices."
- There is no "scientific" style of writing, that is, an approach that automatically provides authenticity and objectivity. In fact, most "scientific writing" is pretentious, often obscure and usually unintelligible. If you think you are writing "scientifically," take a second and critical look at the manuscript.
- Always remember that the report is a scientific treatise. Slang, colloquialisms, and pseudo-scientific jargon should be avoided as much as possible. In fact, repeated use of technical jargon tends to trivialize the subject matter.

- It is acceptable to use abbreviations, for example, DMA instead of dynamic mechanical analysis, provided that you define the abbreviation the first time it is used, for example, "DMA (dynamic mechanical analysis) was used to...."
- Avoid long paragraphs. First, a long paragraph is difficult to read right through without losing track of the beginning. Second, when several facts or concepts are lumped together, they lose impact and this detracts from the value of the work. Consequently, always start a new paragraph for each significant statement or point that is being made. This results in a more readable text and lends greater weight to the subject matter.
- Remember the report is intended for educated and literate readers. There is little need to belabor a point or to repeat the same phrase in several but slightly different ways. If a particular point must be reemphasized, do so in the conclusions which are there for that purpose.
- Follow the basic rules of syntax. Few write perfect English but everyone can try to write grammatically correct English. For example, ensure that verbs agree with their subjects. Also, most word processors now incorporate a grammar check capability. While you might not always agree with the way the grammar checker has corrected the sentence, using the tool may provide a useful guide to correct English when in doubt. Always check the checker by reading through the manuscript after it is completed.
- Double check for spelling errors, missed words, and always make sure that what you have written is what you wanted to write. In other words, does it make sense?
- Do not use dashes or a series of periods to join or link two separate but interrelated phrases into one sentence. Use a semicolon.
- Do not repeat the same word in a sentence or even several times in the same paragraph. Most word processors have a built-in thesaurus (under tools: language) that can be used to avoid this mistake.
- Punctuation is always a problem. When in doubt, I read the sentence out loud (or, more usually, mutter it to myself) and at places where I draw a breath, I insert a comma.
- Finally, it is difficult to write a dissertation or to get a paper into a scientific journal but no one ever got a higher degree, published a scientific paper, or received research funding through a grant application without putting pen to paper.

USEFUL KEYSTROKES FOR WORD

Many commonly used symbols can be found in the "insert" menu of word processors under "symbol" or using keystrokes. For most of the symbols listed below, the "Alt" is held down and the associated number is entered:

Keystroke	Symbol	Application
Alt [24]	↑	Arrow up (increasing)
Alt [25]	↓	Arrow down (decreasing)
Alt [171]	$\frac{1}{2}$	One-half
Alt [224]	α	Greek alpha
Alt [225]	β	Greek beta
Alt [230]	μ	As in microns (μm)
Alt [241]	$\pm$	As in mean $\pm$ standard deviation
Alt [246]	$\div$	Division
Alt [248]	$\circ$	As in 10°C
Alt [250]	·	As in $PdSO_4 \cdot 2H_2O$
Alt [253]	2	As in 10^2 or mm^2
Ctrl C	Copy	Copies a delineated section
Ctrl V	Paste	Pastes the copied section
Ctrl X	Delete	Deletes the delineated section

Using these keystrokes can save a lot of "hunting and pecking" or furious looking through the symbol subfile of insert in the word processor software. It should be noted, however, that symbols entered into the text by a word processor can sometimes change with the text font being used.

A very useful facility in Microsoft Word is the automatic converting of "1/4" to $\frac{1}{4}$, "3/4" to $\frac{3}{4}$, and "1/2" to $\frac{1}{2}$. This is achieved when typing the manuscript by typing in "1", then "/", and finally the "4" and Word automatically makes the conversion. Word will also convert "rd" to rd as in the "3rd quarter." To do this, simply enter the number and then rd followed by a space and the conversion occurs automatically.

One other automatic conversion within Word can be irritating or misleading under certain circumstances, namely the automatic conversion of "(c)" to "©." Consequently, when items of information are presented as a list:

(a). . ...
(b). . ...
(c) . . ...
etc.,

it is sensible to check for this unwanted conversion. One way round this problem is to type in "(c)" and then go back and remove the space between "(" and "c)".

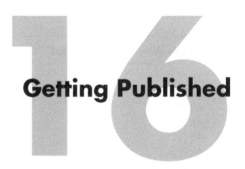

Getting Published

Besides the sense of accomplishment of completing a research study and successfully submitting a dissertation or thesis for a higher degree, one of the most satisfactory endeavors is the submission of a manuscript to a professional journal. The comments made in previous chapters of this book should be useful in this regard, but it has to be stated that mere submission of a manuscript does not guarantee acceptance and publication. Several factors operate here.

MANUSCRIPT REVIEW

The lead author of a scientific paper intended for publication, that is, the manuscript, should read and re-read it to check for scientific accuracy, correct grammar and punctuation, and to ensure that it says what the author intended to say. Waiting a few days before re-reading a manuscript often helps the author to look at it with fresh eyes and see what might have been missed upon first or even second reading. Then, the sensible author will ask one or more colleagues and hopefully his or her mentor to review and possibly edit the manuscript for both content and presentation. The more people who review a manuscript will help in progressively reducing the number of possible errors and other problems remaining within the text. The review of a manuscript by someone who does not have specialized knowledge in that particular area can be very useful in highlighting statements or comments that might appear to be obvious to specialists, particularly the author, but might be less so to others. Of particular importance here is the selection of the correct or the most current terminology. When in doubt, consult terminologies recommended by professional organizations and specialist societies.

Table 16.1 Criteria for successful manuscript submission to journals.

1. Is the science good?
2. Is the manuscript well written?
3. Does the content make a contribution to existing knowledge?
4. Is the manuscript "pitched" at the correct level?
5. Does the manuscript follow the editorial guidelines of the journal?
6. Is the manuscript content in accord with the editorial policy of the journal?
7. Is the literature review comprehensive and up-to-date?

JOURNAL SELECTION

Successful submission of a manuscript to a journal, that is, getting the manuscript accepted by the editorial reviewers and eventually published, requires several criteria to be satisfied, including those indicated in Table 16.1.

The advice and comments of colleagues and mentors are important here since they will suggest suitable venues for manuscripts, but the content of the manuscript must match that of other articles published in the target journal. Whereas it might be intuitively obvious that a manuscript on metallurgy might not be suitable for submission to a dental journal, an article discussing the corrosion of implantable metal alloys in chloride media might have appeal. The proviso here is that the reader should not be expected to deal with a manuscript comprising numerous arcane and very specialized comments on metallurgy or electrochemistry. In other words, authors must ensure that the manuscript and its content are directed to the stated readership and interests of that journal.

Literature citations, that is, calling up of references, in the text must be in accord with journal requirements. Authors who neglect to observe this simple requirement risk summary rejection of their submissions.

MANUSCRIPT SUBMISSION

In the past, multiple copies of manuscripts had to be submitted to journals by regular mail. Now, most journals have established online submission systems which has greatly simplified the process and reduced costs. Further, Assistant and Section Editors usually are glad to help with questions or problems that authors might have with submissions.

Journals generally provide on their web site a section devoted to Instructions for Authors and all authors are strongly encouraged to very carefully review these instructions before submitting a manuscript. Some journals, for example, have strict limitations on the word counts for different categories of articles within that journal. Ignoring these requirements will not elicit a favorable response from reviewers and the Section Editor. Another cause for rejection of a submitted manuscript is poor organization, particularly if the required format has not been followed.

Although it may seem obvious, all authors are advised to check on the recommended font, font style, and size whenever a manuscript submission is to be made. Many journals have a preferred font and organizers of professional meetings commonly have very specific font requirements (and word counts) for submitted abstracts. Ignoring the guidelines can result in summary rejection.

EDITORIAL REVIEW

All journals are good but some are better than others. Thus, it is considered better by one's colleagues (and promotion committees) to be published in a peer-reviewed journal than in one without such editorial review. Likewise, within a given field, some journals are regarded as the premier publications whereas others may rank slightly lower in reputation. It follows that premier journals generally but not always have more rigorous review criteria than others so that getting a manuscript accepted can be challenging with the more prestigious journals.

In this context, it is worth noting that reviewers generally do not like to reject manuscripts out of hand unless of course one or more of the criteria indicated in Table 16.1 are not satisfied. In fact, most reviewers will offer advice to submitting authors on how the manuscript can be improved or at least be brought in line with editorial policy.

The most common grounds for a less than favorable review by editorial reviewers are indicated in Table 16.2.

In many instances an author may be advised to subdivide a very large manuscript into two or more smaller papers so that proper attention can be devoted to all aspects of a study. Likewise, an author may be advised that one aspect of a study covered in a manuscript has been stressed whereas other aspects that were only briefly considered might be equally

Table 16.2 Principal reasons for manuscript rejection.

a. Poor science
b. Bad writing (incorrect syntax, grammar and misleading statements)
c. Content not directed at target audience
d. Nonadherence to editorial policy
e. Content does not contribute to existing knowledge
f. Content poorly organized
g. The literature review is inadequate or incomplete.

as important as, or more interesting than, the primary subject under discussion. Again, the advice of senior colleagues can be very useful in this regard. Remember, most people love to give advice and when that advice can help others, it can be very rewarding.

It is worth mentioning that the average scientist reportedly publishes between 6 and 10 scientific papers throughout his or her career. If you, as a new investigator or even an experienced researcher, can successfully complete a project, write it up and publish it, then you have truly achieved something to be proud of. You have advanced science, added to knowledge, and done something unique because no one has done it before.

Good luck with your research endeavors for they are worth it.

Part II
Statistics and Statistical Analysis

Basic Statistics

According to Mark Twain, Benjamin Disraeli is reported to have said: "There are three types of lies: Lies, Damned Lies and Statistics!" However, problems that arise with statistics are not with the statistics themselves but how they are interpreted. It was Benjamin Franklin who said that "Half the truth is often a great lie."

Regardless of how any researcher feels about statistics, it is virtually impossible to write an acceptable dissertation let alone get a paper published in a reputable journal if the presented data have not been subjected to statistical analysis. It may be safely said that no statistical analysis should be performed unless the answer is intuitively obvious. There is an element of truth to that attitude and one should be wary of manuscripts whose authors have used highly sophisticated analytical tools to prove that there is a minute statistically significant difference in two or more sets of data.

The following chapters present the new researcher, and even the more experienced scientist, with an overview of statistics and statistical analyses. These chapters are not designed to replace the standard statistical textbooks and monographs, many of which are listed as further reading in the Appendix. Nor are they intended to obviate the need to consult a statistician during the planning stages of a project or when analyzing and interpreting the derived data. The intention has been to indicate what should be looked for and how to look for it so that if and when more sophisticated techniques and approaches are required, the researcher knows what questions to address with the statistician of choice. This will save time and avoid much frustration as the project and manuscript near completion.

It should be mentioned that many of the statistical tests discussed in these pages may be performed using the built-in capabilities of spreadsheets, for example, those of Microsoft Excel. Other tests can be performed using readily available statistics packages such as ProStat, StatView, Stat-Lab, and SPSS among others. Where possible, reference will be made to calculations performed with the programs within Excel. Most statistical analysis packages as well as those in Excel will automatically calculate probabilities and indicate significance levels, considerably simplifying preliminary data analyses.

STATISTICS AND STATISTICAL ANALYSIS

A statistic is a single item of information and what in common parlance is commonly known as "statistics" is, in fact, the science of studying data. The correct term for the latter should be statistical analysis. Statistical data and their analysis are central to our lives since they impact many of our decisions, including insurance, education, investments, health care, manufacturing, military spending, and a multitude of others. The function and objective of statistical analysis are to impose order on a disorderly world by looking at what happened, that is, events, and to ask questions such as:

- Was the event an accident or chance occurrence?
- Was the observed effect real?
- Was the observed effect or reaction a coincidence?
- How likely is it that given the same circumstances, the event will happen again?

In other words, statistical analysis predicts the future by looking at the past.

POPULATIONS AND SAMPLES

When data on a group of individuals are collected, for example, heights, weights, or IQs of people or the dimensions, hardnesses, or other parameters of manufactured items, it may be impractical if not impossible to evaluate the entire group, particularly when the groups are large. Further, the composition of the measured group and its characteristics can change on an irregular basis, a common problem when measuring the strength of dental materials which are subject to batch and manipulative variations.

Consequently, rather than trying to measure the tensile strength of every specimen that could be fabricated from the whole day's production of a composite restorative material, that is, making measurements on the entire *population*, a small portion of the population, namely a *sample*, is examined. If the sample is representative of the population, then analysis of the sample data permits conclusions to be drawn, or at least inferred, about the population as a whole. This is known as *inductive statistics* or *statistical inference* but, because the conclusions cannot be stated with absolute certainly, the inferences are stated in terms of *probability*, which is discussed later.

If data derived from a sample are not used to derive an inference or conclusion about the larger group (i.e., the population), the collected data are called *descriptive statistics*.

VARIABLES

A *variable* can assume any value within a set of data whereas a *constant* can have only a single value. A *continuous variable* can (theoretically) assume any value within a range, for example, weights can be 40, 45.2, 48.9 kg, etc., but a *discrete variable* will have a definite value, for example, a patient may have 15, 18, or even 32 teeth but not 20.5 or 30 1/4 or one quarter teeth.

In this context, it is useful to address two other issues, rounding of data and significant figures. It is customary to round numbers containing decimals to the even integer preceding a 5 or to the even integer following a 6: for example, 45.275 is rounded to 45.28 whereas 47.386 is rounded to 47.39; similarly, larger numbers, for example, bacterial counts, are rounded to the nearest million, for example, 114,450,000 is rounded to 114,000,000 or 114×10^6. This practice minimizes *cumulative rounding errors* if multiple calculations must be performed.

In any computation (i.e., addition, subtraction, multiplication, division, and extraction of square roots), the result should not have more significant figures than the numbers with the fewest significant figures, for example, when calculating the value of $A \times B$ in the following spreadsheet, the calculated result must be rounded down to the stated value (Table 17.1); that is, the product of 47.32×29.37 is 1389.79 and the product of 47.32×29.3 is 1386.5.

Because computers express the results of calculations to eight significant places, the unwary will often express their data to the same level of significance. This is shown in the example of calculating square roots in an Excel spreadsheet (Table 17.2) and the stated value of $\sqrt{67.1}$ (or $67.1^{\frac{1}{2}}$) in a report or thesis should be 8.2.

Table 17.1

		$A \times B$	
A	B	Calculated	Stated
47.32	29.37	1389.7884	1389.79
47.32	29.3	1386.4760	1386.5

Table 17.2

C	Square root of C	Stated value
65.37	8.085171612	8.08
67.1	8.191458967	8.2

Another general rule for expressing data is that if measurements are made to one significant place (i.e., one decimal point), then the data should also be restricted to one decimal place. Thus, if dimensions are measured to 0.01 mm, it is incorrect to express surface areas to more than two decimal places. This rule is shown in the following spreadsheet (Table 17.3) and the stated surface area in the report or dissertation should be 25.52.

Table 17.3

Length (mm)	Width (mm)	Calculated Surface area (mm²)	Stated Surface area (mm²)
7.19	3.55	25.5245	25.52

NOTE

In order to perform the statistical tests described in this book, it is necessary to install the *analysis toolpak* in Microsoft Excel since this tool pack provides the functions for performing data analysis.

INSTALLING THE ANALYSIS TOOLPAK

On the *tools* menu, click *add-ins*. In the *add-ins* list, if *analysis toolpak* does not have a check mark, click that box to select it, click *OK*, and then follow the instructions.

USING THE ANALYSIS TOOLPAK

On the *tools* menu, click *data analysis*. In the *data analysis* dialog box, click the name of the analysis tool to be used and then click *OK*. In the dialog box for the selected analytical tool, set the analysis options that are wanted. If in doubt, use the *help* button on the dialog box to get more information on the various options available.

Data and Data Distributions

Collected data that have not been organized are known as *raw data*, and are difficult to evaluate and analyze (Table 18.1). When a series of numbers is placed in ascending (or descending) order or names are ordered alphabetically, the organized data are known as an *array*. Ordering of data is one of the tools that can be used within Excel.

Further, Excel can determine many items of descriptive statistics from these data by highlighting it and following the prompts under *tools: data analysis*. The results are shown in Table 18.2. The meaning and significance of these terms will be discussed later.

For an array or ordered series of numbers, the difference between the minimum and maximum values is known as the *range*. In an array of values or data items, the number of times a particular numeral occurs is known as its *frequency*.

GROUPED DATA

When a large mass of data is summarized, it is useful to place the data into classes or categories and then determine the number of items within each class. For example, when measuring the heights or weights of a group of people, the data would be grouped into classes. Ideally, the data range is divided into a convenient number of classes (*class intervals*) of the same size, but open class intervals are known and used. Further, it simplifies calculations if the *class mark* (midpoint of the class interval) coincides with an actual data item. An example is shown in Table 18.3.

All the people with a weight in the range of 45–49 kg are assumed to have the weight of 47 kg. Mathematical analysis can be used to adjust for small inconsistencies in the data, known as *grouping errors*.

Plotting out the data as a histogram (Figure 18.1) clearly indicates the distribution of the weights.

Table 18.1   Raw and ordered data.

Raw data	Data array
47	36
43	43
73	46
86	47
96	47
47	61
36	62
61	63
46	71
98	73
63	86
71	96
62	98

Table 18.2   Descriptive statistics of the data in Table 18.1.

Mean	63.77
Standard error	5.62
Median	62
Mode	47
Standard deviation	20.28
Sample variance	411.19
Kurtosis	−0.87
Skewness	0.48
Range	62
Minimum	36
Maximum	98
Sum	829
Count	13

Table 18.3   Weights of a group of people.

Weight (kg)	Frequency (number of people)	Class mark
45–49	3	47
50–54	7	52
55–59	10	57
60–64	17	62
65–69	11	67
70–74	6	72
75–79	4	77

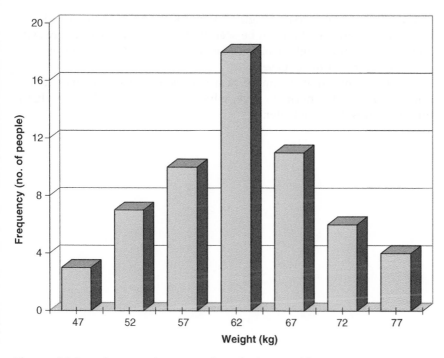

Figure 18.1   Frequency histogram of weight data in Table 18.3.

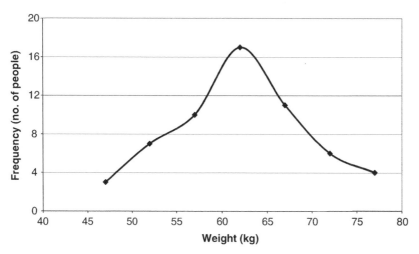

Figure 18.2   Frequency curve of weight data.

If the frequencies versus weight class marks from Table 18.3 are plotted as a curve (Figure 18.2), it can be seen that the data are reasonably symmetrical about the weight of 62 kg. This central value (62 kg) is the average or *mean* weight for the data set.

The most important example of a symmetrical (or bell-shaped) frequency curve is the normal curve, which is critical in probability distributions and is discussed later.

19

Averages (Measures of Central Tendency)

The *average* is the typical or representative value of a set of data and since typical values for an array of numerical data usually lie in the middle of that array, averages are called *measures of central tendency*. There are, however, several types of averages, the most common of which is the *arithmetic mean* or, simply, the *mean* value, denoted by the symbol, $\bar{x}$. Other averages are the *median, mode, geometric mean*, and *harmonic mean* (Table 19.1), and each of these has a different purpose in statistical analysis.

The arithmetic mean is always greater than the geometric mean, which in turn is always greater than the harmonic mean.

MEAN, MEDIAN, AND MODE

If the weekly incomes of five people are $100, $100, $200, $400, and $2,000, the different averages are shown in Table 19.2.

In this example, the values of the mean, median, and mode can be obtained by inspection. However, as noted in Chapter 18, when there are many more values to be determined, one generally has to resort to a computer. Descriptive statistics for the example of five salaries is shown in Table 19.3 and a more complex example is shown in Table 19.4.

Looking at the example of the five salaries in Table 19.2, it is obvious that none of these averages describes the data reasonably and that is the basis for the calculation of other statistics such as standard deviations and standard errors. These are discussed in the next chapter.

GEOMETRIC AND HARMONIC MEANS

The arithmetic mean is based on the assumption that the array of data items increases linearly. This is a reasonable assumption when one is

Table 19.1 Averages.

Type of average	Definition
Arithmetic mean	Representative of a group of observations or values that increase linearly
Median	Center value of a series of observations or values that increase linearly
Mode	Observation that occurs most frequently in a series of values that increase linearly
Geometric mean	Used to calculate average growth rates (e.g., growth of *populations*) or to compound interest for variable interest rates
Harmonic mean	Used to calculate the average of a series of changing *rates*

Table 19.2 Mean, median, and mode for a set of five salaries.

Average	Mean	Median	Mode
Definition	Average income	Middle income	Most common income
Value	$560	$200	$100

Table 19.3 Descriptive statistics of tabulated data using the Excel spreadsheet.

Incomes			
	$100	Mean	$560
	$100	Standard error	$364
	$200	Median	$200
	$400	Mode	$100
	$2,000	Standard deviation	$814
		Sample variance	$663,000
		Range	$1,900
		Minimum	$100
		Maximum	$2,000
		Sum	$2,800
		Count	5

Table 19.4 Descriptive statistics of tabulated data using the Excel spreadsheet.

	100
	200
	350
	400
	400
	425
	450
	575
	650
	725
	850
	875
	935
	1,200
	1,350
	1,425
	1,525
	1,675
	1,750
	1,875
	1,910
	1,950
	2,000
Mean	$1,025.87
Standard error	$131.61
Median	$875.00
Mode	$400.00
Standard deviation	$631.18
Sample variance	$398,383.30
Range	$1,900.00
Minimum	$100.00
Maximum	$2,000.00
Sum	$23,595.00
Count	23

measuring the heights, weights, and intelligence quotients of a group of people. That assumption is not valid when studying the growth of a population because populations tend to follow an exponential rate of increase, that is, an ever-increasing rate of growth.

Consider the case of a city whose total population in 1960 was 250,000. If the population reached 655,000 in 1970, what was the population in

Year	Population	
1960	250,000	
1970	655,000	
Mean	452,500	← ——— =AVERAGE(B2:B3)
Geometric mean	404,660	← ——— =GEOMEAN(B2:B3)

Figure 19.1 Calculation of the mean and geometric mean in Excel.

1965? If the population was assumed to grow linearly, it should have been the mean of 250,000 and 655,000, or 452,500. Since the population grew geometrically, the actual population in 1965 was 404,660. Calculating the geometric mean is straightforward using Excel, one simply writes the following instruction in the target cell: "= GEOMEAN(B2:B3)," where in the spreadsheet B2 is 250,000 and B3 is 655,000. The (arithmetic) mean is given by "= AVERAGE(B2:B3)." These instructions are shown in Figure 19.1.

Similarly, if one wishes to calculate the average rate of cell division in a microbiological study, the difference between the mean value and the actual value (given by the harmonic mean) is quite large, namely 25 for the mean and 19.2 for the harmonic mean (Figure 19.2).

Time (minutes)	Cell division rate (div/sec)	
1	40	
2	30	
3	20	
4	10	
Mean	25	← ——— =AVERAGE(B2:B5)
Harmonic mean	19.20	← ——— =HARMEAN(B2:B5)

Figure 19.2 Calculation of the arithmetic mean and harmonic mean in Excel.

Again, the mean value is calculated from the spreadsheet as "= AVERAGE(B2:B5)," whereas the harmonic mean is calculated as "= HARMEAN(B2:B5)." The difference in the results is attributed to the fact that the arithmetic mean disregards the evidence that the rate of cell division changes minute by minute.

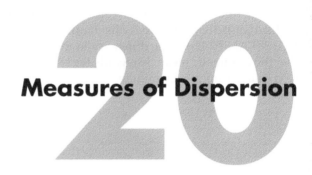

Measures of Dispersion

The *variation* or *dispersion* of numerical data describes their spread about the mean value; common measures of data dispersion are the *range* and the *standard deviation*. Other measures such as mean deviation, semi-interquartile range, and 10–90 percentile range are also used, but standard deviation is used most frequently.

RANGE

The range of a set (array) of numbers is the difference between the largest and smallest numbers in the array. In the set: 2, 4, 4, 7, 7, 7, 10, 11, 12, 14, the range is $14 - 2 = 12$ but may also be expressed as the smallest and largest numbers, for example, 2 to 14 or 2–14.

STANDARD DEVIATION

The *standard deviation*, denoted by the symbol s for a sample and σ for a population, is a measure of the variability or *dispersion* of data about the mean value, $\bar{x}$. A low standard deviation (a small value of s) indicates that the data points are close to the mean, whereas a high standard deviation (a large value of s) indicates a wide spread within the data. An exception to this is when the data follow a bimodal distribution and can have a high standard deviation but actually very little spread. In such cases, the standard deviation might not be an entirely relevant measure.

The standard deviation, commonly abbreviated to S.Dev. or Std. Devn., is expressed in the same units as are the data. The term *standard deviation* has a complex definition, namely it is the square root of the average of the squares of the differences between each datum point and the mean for all

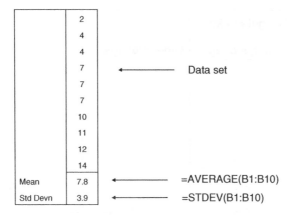

	2	
	4	
	4	
	7	← Data set
	7	
	7	
	10	
	11	
	12	
	14	
Mean	7.8	← =AVERAGE(B1:B10)
Std Devn	3.9	← =STDEV(B1:B10)

Figure 20.1 Calculating the mean and standard deviation using Excel.

data points:

$$s = \sqrt{\frac{[\Sigma(x - \bar{x})^2]}{N}}$$

Fortunately, it is easily calculated using the built-in subroutine within Excel. When the data are entered into a spreadsheet, the mean and standard deviation are readily calculated (Figure 20.1).

The standard deviation also measures confidence in statistical inferences, often expressed as the *margin of error*. In polling data, for example, the reported margin of error is about twice the standard deviation, whereas in finance, the standard deviation in the rate of return on an investment is a measure of the risk. In scientific research, only effects falling outside two or more standard deviations from the mean are considered to be statistically significant.

Standard deviations describe the dispersion of values about their means; however, comparing the dispersions of two sets of data with similar standard deviations but widely different mean values is difficult. An example might be if one wants to compare the relative accuracies of two sets of weights, for example, those of four young children with those of four older siblings. This comparison is possible by calculating the *coefficient of variation* (V or CofV), which is the standard deviation divided by the mean, expressed as a percentage, or $V = (s/\bar{x}) \times 100\%$ (Figure 20.2).

The two coefficients of variation indicate that although the two sets of children were weighed to the precision (±0.5 kg), the relative accuracy (5.7%) in the older sibling weights was about four times greater than that for the younger children (23.5%).

	Weights in kg		
	Young siblings	**Older siblings**	
	2	10.5	
	2.5	11	
	3	11.5	
	3.5	12	
Mean	2.8	11.3 ←	=AVERAGE(B2:B4)
Std. Devn.	0.6	0.6 ←	=STDEV(B2:B4)
Cof V, %	23.5	5.7 ←	= 100*(B7/B6)

Figure 20.2   Means, standard deviations, and coefficients of variation of the weights of younger and older siblings.

The coefficient of variation is a very useful way of comparing the relative accuracies of two or more sets of data. Further, since the coefficient of variation is independent of units, it is useful for comparing distributions based on different units, for example, weights versus heights.

The *variance* of a set of data is the square of the standard deviation, s^2, and is used in statistical testing when comparing the mean values of several sets of data; it is also used by statisticians to correct for the errors caused by grouping data into classes.

STANDARD ERROR OF THE MEAN

The sample mean is commonly used to estimate the population mean but different samples drawn from the same population generally have different mean values. Thus, for example, when the mean strengths of different batches of the same material or component are tested, each set of measurements will have a slightly different mean and standard deviation. Such differences are compounded when small group samples (i.e., $N \leq 30$) or when samples containing different numbers of specimens are measured. If the sample size is increased, the standard deviations will still fluctuate with different samples but each will be a more accurate estimate of the standard deviation of the population. As the sample sizes increase, the sample means can estimate the population mean more accurately.

The standard deviation assesses the variability or dispersion in the measured data but in most situations, the true value of the standard deviation is not known. The term *standard error*, however, refers to an estimate of this unknown quantity. The *standard error of the mean*, SE_{mean} or $SE(\bar{x})$, is the standard deviation of sample means over the samples from the population.

The standard error of the mean is calculated as the standard deviation of a sample divided by the square root of the sample size, N: $SE(\bar{x}) = s/\sqrt{N}$ and measures the precision with which the population mean can be estimated from a sample mean. Larger sample sizes result in more accurate estimates of the population mean and, consequently, the standard error of the mean becomes smaller. Descriptive statistics calculated in Excel will indicate the standard error (see Table 18.2).

In summary, the standard deviation and coefficient of variation indicate the variation among individual observations, whereas the standard error indicates the accuracy of the estimate of the mean. It is unnecessary in a scientific paper or a dissertation to report both the standard error of the mean and the standard deviation since, if the sample size (N) is given together with either the SE or the S.Dev., then the other parameter can be readily calculated.

Standard error is also useful when considering regression, that is, evaluating the variation of a dependent variable (Y) as it relates to an independent variable (X), for example, the variation in patient weights with heights. Excel permits the determination of the standard error of the predicted value of Y for each value of X. This is discussed again in Chapter 23.

Probability and the Normal Curve

Probability theory is central to statistics and contributes to the understanding of the random factors behind almost everything. It is the basis for such diverse entities as weather forecasting, drug interactions and effectiveness, stock market investing, and gambling.

Probability is based on the following two premises:

- An event that has an absolute certainty of occurring has a probability (P) of 100% or $P = 1.0$.
- An event that cannot occur has a probability of 0.0% or $P = 0.0$.

Therefore, the probability of occurrence of all other events lies between 0.0 and 1.0, inclusive, and this is the basis of all statistical testing.

For convenience, statisticians adopt the following criteria:

- If an event such as the difference between two sets of data has a 5% or less chance of occurrence, that is, $P \leq 0.05$, it is said to be *probably significant*. This means that the difference between the data could have occurred by chance only once if the experiment were to be repeated 20 times.
- If an event such as the difference between two sets of data has a 1% or less chance of occurrence, that is, $P \leq 0.01$, it is said to be *significant*. This means that the observed difference between the data could have occurred by chance only once if the experiment were to be repeated 100 times.
- If an event such as the difference between two sets of data has a 0.1% or less chance of occurrence, that is, $P \leq 0.001$, it is said to be *highly significant*. This means that the observed difference between the data sets could have occurred by chance only once if the experiment were to be repeated 1,000 times.

EXPECTATION

Expectation (E) is the expected number of occurrences of an event. It is calculated as the product of the number of trials (the number of times something is performed) and the probability of a successful outcome, $E =$ number of trials, $N \times$ probability, $P = N \times P$.

If the probability of getting "heads" when flipping a coin is 0.5, that is, there is a 50% probability of getting heads with every flip of the coin, then one would expect to get heads 50 times if a coin is flipped 100 times:

$$E_{\text{heads}} = 100 \times 0.5 = 50$$

Expectations can be calculated for most things, for example, the number of times a pair of sixes will come up when two dice are tossed and so on, provided the probability of each event is known or can be surmised. The chance of getting a 6 with a single toss of a die is 1 in 6 or $1/6$ ($P = 0.167$), etc.

THE NORMAL CURVE

Collected data belong to a sample drawn from a much larger population. If those data are continuous, for example, patient weights, etc., and the class intervals are very small, each class would contain appreciable numbers of data points for a population, and unlike Figure 18.2, the *frequency curve* (or probability distribution) would be continuous. As stated above, the most important continuous probability distribution is the one-peaked (unimodal) *normal curve*, also known as the Gaussian curve (Figure 21.1). The total area under the curve is 1.0, which means that the probability of any observation or measurement in a population lying under this curve is $P = 1$ or 100%. The concept of probability forms the basis of all statistical testing.

The peak of the curve occurs at the mean value, and the mean, mode, and median all coincide at the peak. The curve is completely defined by the mean and the standard deviation; the mean of a population is symbolized by μ (compared to $\bar{x}$ for a sample) and the standard deviation by σ (compared to s for a sample). Although the curve can extend to infinity, the normal curve is usually limited to 3 (or sometimes 4) standard deviations.

The area under the curve from $\mu - \sigma$ to $\mu + \sigma$ (i.e., the mean ± 1 standard deviation) encompasses 68.26% of the total area. The area corresponding to $\mu \pm 2\sigma$ encompasses 95.45% and the area for $\mu \pm 3\sigma$ is 99.73%. Thus, 99.73% or 9,973 of 10,000 observations of a population will be found within the range of three standard deviations of the mean.

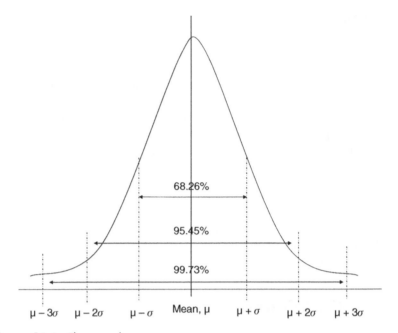

Figure 21.1 The normal curve.

All normal curves have the same property, so despite the fact that two curves may have different values of the mean and standard deviation (Figure 21.2), the percentage of total area within 1, 2, or 3 standard deviations is same for both curves.

The horizontal axis (the abscissa or x-axis) represents the value of the parameter being measured, whereas the vertical axis (the ordinate or y-axis) represents the number of occurrences or frequency.

NORMAL DEVIATE

While the shape of the normal curve is standardized, the scale of plotting the graph determines the height of the peak and the spread of the base. It is possible to convert all normal curves, that is, regardless of the individual values of μ and σ, to a standard or *unit normal curve*. For example, if the values of x represent patient weights, each weight (x value) can be expressed as a deviation from the mean and this value is the *normal deviate*, z:

$$z = \frac{(x - \mu)}{\sigma}$$

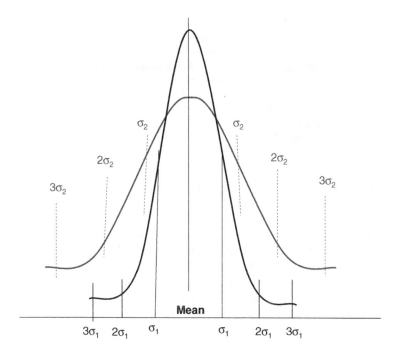

Figure 21.2 Shapes of normal curves with different means and standard deviations.

If all x values are converted to deviations from the mean, the plot of the measurements will have a mean of $\bar{x}$ and a standard deviation of 1. Thus, all normal curves regardless of individual μ and σ values can be transformed into unit normal curves. Further, most statistics textbooks provide tables that give the area under the unit normal curve for different values of z.

The area under the curve between two values of z represents the probability that any randomly selected measurement or parameter will fall between the two z values. An example shows the usefulness of this manipulation: what is the probability of a randomly selected person having an intelligence quotient (IQ) in the range of 90–130 when the mean or average IQ is 100 and the standard deviation is 12?

Converting the x values (the two IQ scores):

$$Z_{IQ90} = \frac{(90 - 100)}{12} = -0.833 \text{ and } Z_{IQ130} = \frac{(130 - 100)}{12} = 2.5$$

and a table of areas under the unit normal curve indicates that 0.7905 (or 79.05%) of the curve lies between these two values, -0.83 to 2.5. It can be concluded that 79% of the population would have an IQ within the range

Table 21.1 Areas under the unit normal curve for different ranges of z values.

Z range	Area under curve (%)
-1 to $+1$	68.26
-1.96 to $+1.96$	95
-2.0 to $+2.0$	95.45
-3.0 to $+3.0$	99.73

of 90–130. Conversely, 21% of the population will have an IQ of less than 90 or greater than 130.

The tabulated areas under the unit normal curve indicate that 68.26% of the area lies between $Z = -1$ and $Z = 1$ and this area, together with those for other ranges of z values, are indicated in Table 21.1.

The areas under the unit normal curve indicate that one can be 95% confident of finding the measured variate between the limits $z = -1.96$ to $z = 1.96$. Further, the values given by $\mu - 1.96\sigma$ and $\mu + 1.96\sigma$ are known as the *95% confidence limits* for the data. The factors or multipliers of σ (e.g., 1, 1.96, 2, 2.58, etc.) are termed the *confidence coefficients* or *critical values* denoted by z_c.

Normal distribution tables are also available, which give the probability of a variate having a z value greater than the selected value. Figure 21.3 indicates the difference between the two derived areas.

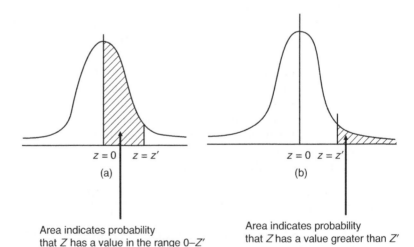

(a) $z = 0$ $z = z'$

Area indicates probability that Z has a value in the range 0–Z'

(b) $z = 0$ $z = z'$

Area indicates probability that Z has a value greater than Z'

Figure 21.3 (a) Area for $z = 0$ and $z = z'$; (b) area for $z > z'$.

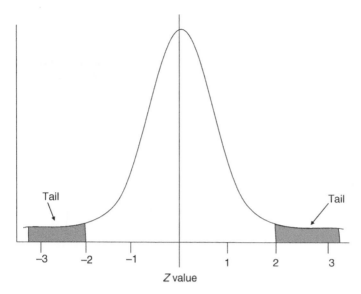

Figure 21.4   Tails of the unit normal distribution.

Finally, the areas to the extreme right or extreme left of the curve are known as the *tails* (Figure 21.4) and are important in statistical testing. In scientific work, only values that lie in the tails are considered to be statistically significant. Many scientists will omit outliers, that is, datum points that are more than two standard deviations from the mean, when presenting data. Such omissions are often justifiable provided that it is clearly stated that outliers have been omitted.

KURTOSIS

In some cases, a slight bias (whether intrinsic or extrinsic to the data) may distort the distribution of the observed data. For instance, grade inflation may result in a greater number of "A"s and "B"s than would be predicted by a strictly normal curve. To compensate, additional parameters such as "skewness," "kurtosis," etc. may be necessary to fit the observed data to a normal curve. These refinements are not uncommon and should not be viewed as data manipulation.

The terms *kurtosis* and *skewness* were introduced in Table 18.2; both terms indicate the shape of the data distribution or frequency curve. Kurtosis is the degree of peakedness of a distribution relative to a normal distribution. Kurtosis is zero for a normal curve (a *mesokurtic* distribution)

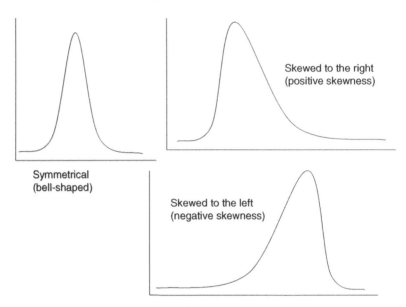

Figure 21.5 Characteristic shapes of distribution curves.

and kurtosis is positive for a *leptokurtic distribution*, the curve of which has a relatively high peak. A *platykurtic* distribution has a flat-topped or relatively unpeaked curve and a negative kurtosis.

The skewness of a distribution curve indicates the asymmetry of the distribution curve (Figure 21.5). The normal curve is symmetrical but the curve is asymmetrical if one tail is longer than the other. The curve is skewed to the right, that is, has *positive skewness*, when the longer tail is to the right whereas if the longer tail is to the left, the curve is skewed to the left and has *negative skewness*.

OTHER DISTRIBUTIONS

Data commonly follow a normal distribution but other distributions of data are known, including the *binomial* (or Bernoulli) distribution and the *Poisson* distribution. The mathematical definitions of these distributions differ from that of the normal distribution.

The binomial distribution describes the probability that an event will occur an exact number of times in a given number of trials, for example, the number of "heads" when flipping a coin a certain number of times. In the binomial distribution, if the sample size N is large, the probability of occurrence of an event (e.g., all "heads" in coin flipping) is close to zero, that is, it is a rare event. With large values of N, the normal distribution closely approximates the binomial distribution. Likewise, the Poisson distribution approaches a normal distribution with large sample sizes. Readers interested in learning more about these distributions should consult the supplemental texts suggested in the Appendix.

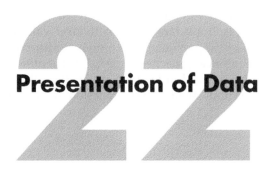

Presentation of Data

Presenting data in an orderly manner is essential both for clarity and for conveying the message regarding its importance and relevance. Although journals, in their zeal to cut publication costs, dislike data being presented in both tabular and graphical forms within the same article, this restriction does not apply to dissertations and reports. In fact, histograms with appropriate standard deviations included as tie bars considerably aid in understanding the data.

Consider as an example the weights of four groups of high school students with ten students in each group. The data are presented in Table 22.1.

Inspection of the data suggests that there are differences between the groups, but how does one show these differences?

If the data are plotted as a histogram with the scale of the ordinate (the weight axis) extending from 0 to 50 (Figure 22.1), the differences although present are not obvious.

If, however, the same data are plotted with a restricted ordinate scale then differences become more apparent (Figure 22.2).

Since this technique can be used by unscrupulous scientists to deceive, an axis break (denoted by zigzag lines on the y-axis) will fully disclose your graphical manipulations.

Although Figure 22.2 suggests differences between the four groups, it does not indicate the dispersion of weights within each group. This is achieved by using *tie bars* which have the values of the standard deviations and are superimposed on the columns representing mean weights (Figure 22.3).

Showing tie bars is quite simple in Excel. After calculating the mean values and their standard deviations in the spreadsheet (Table 22.1), a histogram is plotted using the graphical function in Excel. Then after the histogram is presented/obtained with the appropriate vertical and horizontal axes and all other presentation criteria are satisfactory (i.e., font size,

Table 22.1 Weights of high school students.

Groups	A	B	C	D
	34.09	31.82	32.73	34.09
	36.36	33.18	33.18	36.36
	36.82	34.09	33.64	36.82
	37.27	35.45	34.09	36.82
	37.73	36.36	34.09	37.73
	40.91	37.27	35.91	38.64
	41.82	37.73	35.91	39.09
	42.27	38.18	36.36	39.55
	43.64	38.64	37.27	40.00
	44.55	41.36	37.27	41.36
	46.36	41.82	37.73	41.82
	46.82	43.18	38.64	43.18
Mean	40.7	37.4	35.6	38.8
S.Dev.	4.2	3.5	2.0	2.6
CofV, %	10.3	9.4	5.5	6.7

bold or regular type face etc.), if one places the cursor of the mouse on a column and right clicks, a box will open with "format data series" at the top. Clicking on this opens the box (Figure 22.4). Once open, the style of tie bar can be selected and the values of standard deviations are inserted by clicking on the custom box and inserting the calculated S.Dev. values from Table 22.1. Once "OK" is clicked, Excel does the rest.

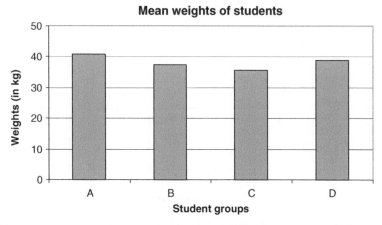

Figure 22.1 Histogram of mean high school student weights.

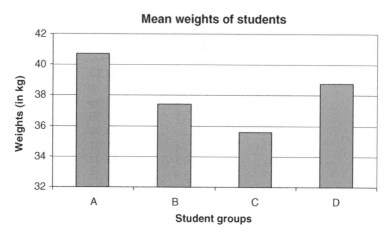

Figure 22.2 Histogram of mean high school student weights with constricted ordinate scale.

The use of tie bars to indicate graphically the dispersion in the data is very useful when a group of data contains outliers, that is, datum points that are two or more standard deviations from the mean (Table 22.2 and Figure 22.5).

Although it can be seen from Table 22.2 that there is a greater dispersion of the weights for Group C students, as shown by the larger standard deviation and coefficient of variation, the histogram in Figure 22.5 makes the differences between groups more obvious. Based on the observed

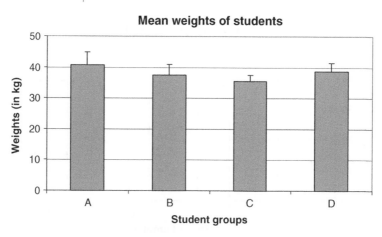

Figure 22.3 Histogram of mean high school student weights with tie bars showing the standard deviations.

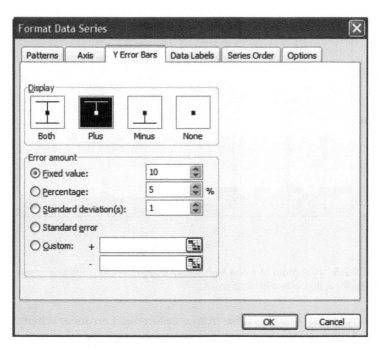

Figure 22.4 Format data series box in Excel.

differences, a statistical test to determine whether differences in the data actually exist would be justified and probably necessary.

If the 60 kg outlier in Group C is eliminated because it is more than two standard deviations from the mean (Table 22.3), then the standard deviation of the group (and the tie bar in the histogram) is reduced (Figure 22.6).

If outliers, that is, datum points that are more than 2 standard deviations from the mean, have been omitted from the data, such action must

Table 22.2 Mean student weights with standard deviations.

Group	Student weights
A	39.6 ± 2.9 (7.3%)
B	37.4 ± 3.5 (9.4%)
C	37.3 ± 7.3 (19.6%)
D	38.8 ± 2.6 (6.7%)

Coefficients of variation are in parentheses.

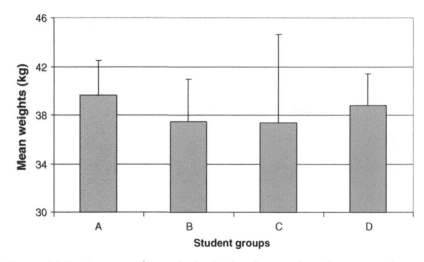

Figure 22.5 Histogram of mean high school student weights with one group having a greater dispersion within its data points.

be clearly stated. Outliers arise from measurement errors or when the observed datum point is clearly out of synchrony with the other members of a group of measurements. However, care must be taken when data are eliminated because even though a datum point might appear to be an aberration, it still counts as data. Consultation with a statistician is advisable in such cases.

Table 22.3 Student weights with and without elimination of the outlier in Group C.

Groups	A	B	C	D	Groups	A	B	C	D
	35.20	31.82	32.73	34.09		35.20	31.82	32.73	34.09
	36.36	33.18	33.18	36.36		36.36	33.18	33.18	36.36
	36.82	34.09	33.64	36.82		36.82	34.09	33.64	36.82
	37.27	35.45	34.09	36.82		37.27	35.45	34.09	36.82
	37.73	36.36	34.09	37.73		37.73	36.36	34.09	37.73
	39.30	37.27	35.91	38.64		39.30	37.27	35.91	38.64
	40.10	37.73	35.91	39.09		40.10	37.73	35.91	39.09
	41.10	38.18	36.36	39.55		41.10	38.18	36.36	39.55
	42.20	38.64	37.27	40.00		42.20	38.64	37.27	40.00
	42.70	41.36	37.27	41.36		42.70	41.36	37.27	41.36
	43.00	41.82	37.73	41.82		43.00	41.82	37.73	41.82
	43.50	43.18	60.00	43.18		43.50	43.18		43.18
Mean	39.6	37.4	37.3	38.8	Mean	39.6	37.4	35.3	38.8
S.Dev.	2.9	3.5	7.3	2.6	S.Dev.	2.9	3.5	1.8	2.6
CofV, %	7.3	9.4	19.6	6.7	CofV, %	7.3	9.4	5.1	6.7

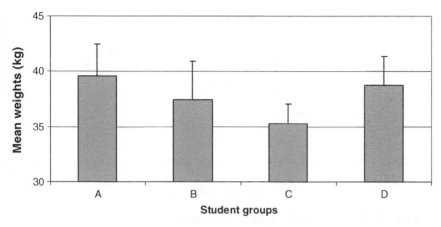

Figure 22.6 Histogram of mean high school student weights with the outlier in Group Comitted.

Data presentation becomes very important when plotting the relationship between a dependent variable and an independent variable, for example, weights against heights. Table 22.4 shows the heights and weights of a group of students. As expected, as student height increases, the weights also increase, as shown in Figure 22.7. However, because some taller students may be lighter than shorter students (and vice versa), a plot of the data appears to contain some "doubling back."

Table 22.4 Student heights and corresponding weights.

Height (cm)	Weight (kg)
144.8	34.1
142.2	36.4
147.3	36.8
149.9	37.3
147.3	37.7
152.4	40.9
152.4	45.0
157.5	42.3
162.6	43.6
172.7	44.5
167.6	49.0
170.2	46.8

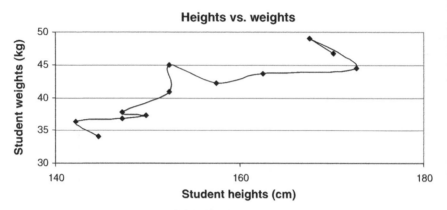

Figure 22.7 Plot of student heights versus weights.

In such cases, it is better to plot the data as a scattergram and then add a trend line as shown in Figure 22.8. This again is a task easily performed in Excel. After the data have been plotted as separate points rather than connected by lines, right click onto the data. When the format data series box comes up, click on add trend line and Excel performs the requisite calculations.

The advantage of adding a trend line is that the plot clearly shows that there is not a precise correlation between heights and weights, for example, some students are lighter than might be expected while others are heavier. The trend line, however, indicates that generally, weights do increase with height in a linear manner but not precisely. This subject will be revisited when discussing regression analysis.

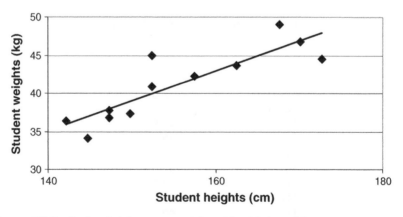

Figure 22.8 Student heights versus weights with added trend line.

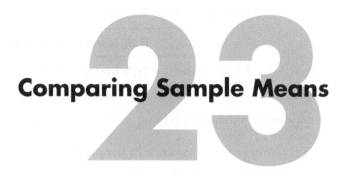

Comparing Sample Means

The most common statistical tests are the ones designed to decide whether the difference between two means could have arisen by chance. Before discussing this, some terminology and factors related to statistical testing must be reviewed.

TERMINOLOGY

The *null hypothesis* (H_0) is the assumption by the observer, the person making the measurements, that there is no difference between two sets of data. If the difference could have arisen by chance, then H_0 can be accepted as *true*. If the difference could not have arisen by chance, then H_0 is *false* and it can be assumed that there is a difference between the two data sets. In this case, the *alternative hypothesis* (H_1), namely that there is a difference between the two data sets, is adopted.

The procedure then is to calculate the probability that the two sets of data are part of the same population. If this probability is less than 5% ($P \leq 0.05$), then the chance that there is no difference between the two data sets (namely that H_0 is true) is less than 1 in 20. In which case, H_0 can be rejected and the alternative hypothesis (H_1) can be accepted.

Although a probability level of 5% is common, some researchers are very cautious and prefer to set higher probability levels, $P \leq 0.01$ or $P \leq 0.001$, before claiming statistically significant differences between data sets.

DEGREES OF FREEDOM

The number of *degrees of freedom* (df or v) of a statistic is defined as the number of independent observations in the sample (N) minus the number

Table 23.1 Errors in hypothesis testing.

	If H_0 is true	If H_0 is false
If H_0 is rejected	**Type I error**	No error
If H_0 is accepted	No error	**Type II error**

of population parameters (k) that must be estimated from sample observations, or $df = N - k$.

This concept can be explained by the paradigm of four people traveling in a four-seater car. One person has to drive but the other travelers, the second, third, and fourth persons, can all pick seats; thus, $k = 1$ since one parameter is fixed. Accordingly, the degrees of freedom will be $df = N - k = 4 - 1 = 3$.

Degrees of freedom are taken into consideration with most statistical tests.

ERRORS IN TESTING

Mention should be made of errors in hypothesis testing as shown in Table 23.1.

Rejection of a null hypothesis when, in fact, it is true is known as a *Type I error*. If the null hypothesis is false but H_0 is accepted, a *Type II error* has been committed. The probability of committing a Type I error is given by α, the specified significance level adopted when performing the statistical test. An $\alpha = 0.05$ is commonly considered to be a small enough chance of committing a Type I error but not so small that there is a large chance of a Type II error.

The probability of committing a Type II error (β) is not known and cannot be specified although it is inversely related to the value of α. Thus, a lower probability of committing a Type I error is associated with a higher probability of a Type II error. Both types of error can be reduced simultaneously by increasing N, the sample size.

Ideally, the null hypothesis, the alternative hypothesis, and the significance level should all be decided upon prior to data collection. The preselected level of significance is known as an *a priori* α.

ONE-TAILED AND TWO-TAILED TESTS

In formulating a hypothesis, two questions can be asked:

(1) Is there a difference between two means or between the mean of a sample ($\bar{x}$) and the population mean (μ)?

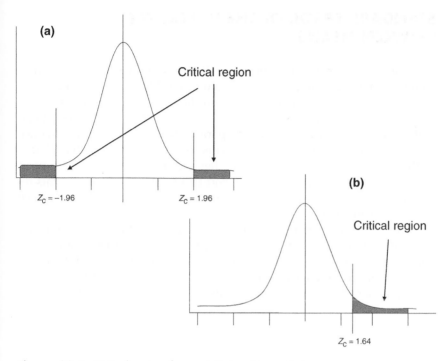

Figure 23.1 Critical regions for one-tailed and two-tailed tests.

(2) Is the mean of a sample ($\bar{x}$) significantly greater (or less) than the population mean (μ)?

Question 1 disregards whether $\bar{x}$ is larger or smaller than μ; the question being asked is whether one material or procedure is different from another. In contrast, question 2 addresses the relative magnitude of $\bar{x}$ compared to μ or mean $\bar{x}_1$ compared to mean $\bar{x}_2$; and the question typically being asked is whether one process or material is better than the other.

With question 1, the critical region for a significance level of $P \leq 0.5$ is equally divided between the two tails such that 2.5% of the area under the curve is in the region at $Z_c < -1.96$ and 2.5% of the area of the curve lies in the region at $Z_c > 1.96$ (Figure 23.1a).

With question 2, the critical region is confined to one tail, which occupies 5% of the area under the curve and for this probability, $Z_c > 1.64$ (Figure 23.1b).

The consequence of this is that a given score of a normal deviate has a higher probability in a one-tailed test than in a two-tailed test, which affects significance levels in statistical testing.

STANDARD ERROR OF THE DIFFERENCE BETWEEN MEANS

The standard error qualifies the mean. If two or more series of measurements are made on samples drawn from ostensibly the same population, there always will be small differences in the means of each series due to differences in sampling. Nevertheless, departures from the overall mean that exceed 2 standard errors are comparatively rare, occurring about once in every 20 trials or 5% of the time. This stems from the fact that 95.45% of the area under the normal curve lies within the range of the mean ± 2 standard errors (see Chapter 21 and Figure 21.1); accordingly, this relationship can be used to test the statistical significance of the difference between means (Figure 23.2).

Consider the case of a series of N_1 measurements that were made and which were found to have a mean $\bar{x}_1$ and standard deviation s_1, and a second series of N_2 measurements with a mean $\bar{x}_2$ and a standard deviation s_2. The variances of the two series are $s_1{}^2/N_1$ and $s_2{}^2/N_2$, or $(SE\bar{x}_1)^2$ and $(SE\bar{x}_2)^2$, where the variance is simply the square of the standard deviation, $var = s^2$.

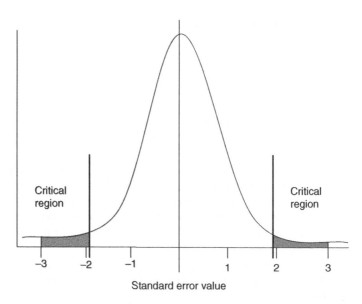

Critical region

Critical region

Standard error value

Figure 23.2 Critical regions for significance ($P \leq 0.05$): the sample lies outside the range of -1.96 to 1.96.

The variance of the sum or difference of two independent random samples is equal to the sum of their variances so that

$$\text{Variance of difference between means} = (\text{SE}\bar{x}_1)^2 + (\text{SE}\bar{x}_2)^2$$

The standard error of the difference between means is the square root of the variance of the difference between means, or

$$\text{SE of difference between means} = \sqrt{[(\text{SE}\bar{x}_1)^2 + (\text{SE}\bar{x}_2)^2]}$$

If the observed difference between the two means is more than twice the standard error of the difference between means, this difference is "probably significant." Thus, if

$$[\bar{x}_1 - \bar{x}_2] \geq 2 \times \left[\sqrt{(\text{SE}\bar{x}_1)^2 + (\text{SE}\bar{x}_2)^2}\right], \; P < 0.05$$

This is best shown by an example in which the diametral tensile strengths ascertained in a series of ten determinations are compared (Figure 23.3).

	DTS measurements	
	A	**B**
	28.0	24.0
	28.5	24.5
	29.0	25.0
	30.0	25.9
	30.7	26.0
	30.8	26.2
	31.0	27.0
	32.0	27.3
	33.0	28.0
	34.0	29.5
Mean	30.7	26.3	=AVERAGE(B3:B12)
S.Dev.	1.9	1.7	=STDEV(B3:B12)
SE	0.6	0.5	=B14/(N^0.5)
Difference between means:	4.4	← =B13-C13
Variance of difference between means:	0.7	← =(B14^2) + (C14^2)
SE of difference between means:	0.8	← =B17^0.5
Ratio	5.4	

Figure 23.3 Calculation of the standard error of the difference between means in Excel (Excel spreadsheet instructions are indicated).

	A	B		
	28.0	24.0		
	28.5	24.5		
	29.0	25.0		
	30.0	25.9		
	30.7	26.0		
	30.8	26.2		
	31.0	27.0		
	32.0	27.3		
	33.0	28.0		
	34.0	29.5		
Mean	30.7	26.3	←	=AVERAGE(B3:B12)
S.Dev.	1.9	1.7	←	=STDEV(B3:B12)
Variance	3.7	2.8	←	=B14^2

Figure 23.4 Organization of data for performing z-test: two sample for means in Excel (Excel spreadsheet instructions are indicated).

The calculation shows that the difference between the two means (4.4) is more than five times greater than the standard error of the difference between means (0.8), a difference that is considerably greater than 2 standard errors. It can be concluded that there is a statistically significant difference between the strengths of the two materials.

The standard error of the difference between means can be used to determine whether the observed difference in mean values is statistically significant. However, the calculations are somewhat tedious and have to be performed "manually" by writing instructions into the Excel spreadsheet. Fortunately, Excel incorporates software that performs the same calculation although the data still have to be manipulated slightly in order to satisfy the input required for the calculation.

Considering the data in Figure 23.3, the variances (the squares of the standard deviations) must be calculated as shown in Figure 23.4.

Thereafter, under the drop-down menu *tools: data analysis*, select *z-test: two sample for means*. Follow the prompts for data entry, noting that the hypothesized difference between means is 0 and the variable 1 variance will be 3.7 and the variable 2 variance will be 2.8. Excel will then calculate the z-test statistic, the critical values of z for one- and two-tailed tests and the probabilities of there being a statistically significant difference between the two mean values (Table 23.2).

The advantage of using Excel for determining whether there is a statistically significant difference between means is that the significance level

Table 23.2 Excel calculation of the z-score for the difference between two means.

z-Test: two sample for means		
	Material A	**Material B**
Mean	30.7	26.3
Known variance	3.7	1.7
Observations	10	10
Hypothesized mean difference	0	
z	5.933	
$P(Z \leq z)$ one-tailed	1.49×10^{-9}	
$z_{critical}$ one-tailed	1.645	
$P(Z \leq z)$ two-tailed	2.97×10^{-9}	
$z_{critical}$ two-tailed	1.960	

(α) can be specified and that the program calculates the probabilities of there being a real (statistically significant) difference between the means.

A more convenient approach to making such a comparison is to use Student's t-test, a statistical method that is built into Excel. This test is discussed in Chapter 24.

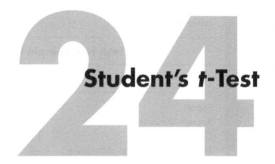

Student's *t*-Test

The use of the standard error of the mean to test the significance of the difference between two means was discussed in Chapter 23. Another test widely used for this purpose, and one that is computationally simpler because it is built into Excel, is Student's *t*-test. This test involves the *t* distribution, discovered by Gosset, a mathematician who used the pseudonym "Student."

COMPARING A SAMPLE WITH A UNIVERSAL MEAN

In many studies, the mean of a sample ($\bar{x}$) of N values is compared with that of the population from which it is drawn, where the population has a mean μ and a variance σ^2. If repeated independent samples were taken from the same population, the samples should be normally distributed around the population mean μ and the standardized variate z can be used to determine the *probability* that the observed mean ($\bar{x}$) significantly differs from μ:

$$ Z = \frac{\bar{x} - \mu}{\text{SE}(\mu)} = \frac{(\bar{x} - \mu)}{\sigma/\sqrt{N}} = \frac{(\bar{x} - \mu)}{\sigma} \times \sqrt{N} $$

However, the standard deviation of the population (σ) is generally not known and, consequently, the normal deviate (z) cannot be calculated. This problem can be avoided by using the sample variance (s^2) in place of σ^2 and calculating the *t*-statistic:

$$ t = \frac{\bar{x} - \mu}{s/\sqrt{N}} = \frac{(\bar{x} - \mu)}{s} \times \sqrt{N} $$

$$\text{where } t = \frac{\text{Difference between means}}{\text{Estimated standard error of the mean}}$$

In other words, the standard deviation of the population is estimated from the sample standard deviation s, which is performed using the relation:

$$s^2 = \frac{\Sigma(x - \bar{x})^2}{N - 1}$$

Thus, the statistic t is computed in the same way as the normal deviate z but using s in place of σ. There is one major difference between the statistics z and t, namely that while there is only one standard normal curve (i.e., when using the z-statistic), there is a family of t curves corresponding to each degree of freedom. The t curves are very similar to the normal curve, particularly with large degrees of freedom ($df \geq 30$), so that t values are very similar to the corresponding z values of the normal distribution when samples with a large N are studied.

Statistics textbooks have tabulated values of t for different probabilities and degrees of freedom. Conveniently, when the value of the t-statistic is calculated using Excel, the spreadsheet will also indicate the critical value of t (t_c) for significance and the probability for both a one-tailed and a two-tailed test.

COMPARISON OF TWO MEANS USING THE *t*-TEST

In many situations, there may not be a standard to which the sample can be compared and, more commonly, a researcher has two sets of data and wants to compare them to determine whether there is a real difference between them. Therefore, the question being asked is whether the difference between the two groups has arisen from sampling variation (the null hypothesis) or due to a real difference between the means (the alternative hypothesis). For Groups A and B with means $\bar{x}_A$ and $\bar{x}_B$ and standard deviations s_A and s_B, the t-statistic is calculated as:

$$t = \frac{\bar{x}_A - \bar{x}_B}{\sqrt{[s^2(1/N_A + 1/N_B)]}}$$

where s^2 is known as the *pooled variance* and is calculated from s_A and s_B by:

$$s^2 = \frac{(N_A - 1) \times s_A^2 + (N_B - 1) \times S_B^2}{N_A + N_B - 2}$$

Table 24.1 Diametral strength test (DTS) performed on two restorative materials (strengths in MPa).

	Material A	**Material B**
	28.0	24.0
	28.5	24.5
	29.0	25.0
	30.0	25.9
	30.7	26.0
	30.8	26.2
	31.0	27.0
	32.0	27.3
	33.0	28.0
	34.0	29.5
Mean	30.7	26.3
S.Dev.	1.9	1.7
CofV, %	6.3	6.3

The calculated t value follows Student's t distribution with $(N_A - 1) + (N_B - 1) = N_A + N_B - 2$ degrees of freedom.

The use of the t-test can be demonstrated by looking again at the two sets of diametral strength test values (Table 24.1), which were mixed, stored, and tested under identical conditions.

Inspection of the data indicates that the data for the two materials have equal variances (i.e., very similar standard deviations). Although inspection of the coefficients of variation clearly indicates equality of the variances, in many instances with more complex data sampling, equality of variances should be confirmed with the *variance ratio test* (the F-test) prior to performing a t-test. In Excel, under *tools: data analysis*, click on *F-test two-sample for variances*. Follow the data entry prompts and the F ratio is automatically calculated (Table 24.2).

Table 24.2 F-test for two-sample variances.

	Material A	**Material B**
Mean	30.7	26.3
Variance	3.7	2.8
Observations	10	10
df	9	9
F	1.335	
$P(F \leq f)$ one-tailed	0.337	
$F_{critical}$ one-tailed	3.179	

Table 24.3 Calculated *t*-statistics and corresponding probabilities for differences between means.

	Material A	Material B
Mean	30.7	26.3
Variance	3.7	2.8
Observations	10	10
Pooled variance	3.25	
Hypothesized mean difference	0	
df	18	
t-statistic	5.40	
$P(T \le t)$ one-tailed	0.000	
$t_{critical}$ one-tailed	1.73	
$P(T \le t)$ two-tailed	3.9×10^{-5}	
$t_{critical}$ two-tailed	2.10	

The calculated data indicate that the value of F is significantly less than the critical value of F ($F_{critical}$) for a significant difference between the two variances and the probability of a difference is $P = 0.34$, that is, considerably greater than $P < 0.05$. It can be concluded that there is no difference in the variances of the two samples and, accordingly, the *t*-test to be performed will be based on *two-sample t-test assuming equal variances* in Excel.

For this, select *t-test: two-sample assuming equal variances* under *tools: data analysis* and enter the data as prompted. Excel will then calculate the *t*-statistic and indicate the critical value of *t* (t_c) for both a one-tailed test and a two-tailed test together with the corresponding probabilities of a difference between the two mean values (Table 24.3).

Since the calculated *t*-statistic (5.40) is markedly greater than t_c (1.73 for a one-tailed test and 2.10 for a two-tailed test), it may be concluded that the difference between the two means is statistically significant. The calculated probability of a difference is $P = 0.000$ for a one-tailed test and $P = 3.9 \times 10^{-5}$ for a two-tailed test.

If the variances for the two samples are unequal (Table 24.4), a modified *t*-test must be performed.

The *F*-ratio test confirms, as surmised from the coefficients of variation, that the variances of the two sets of data are different (Table 24.5).

Since the two data sets have unequal variances, under the drop-down menu *tools: data analysis*, select *t-test: two-sample assuming unequal variances* and enter the appropriate data, and Excel will calculate the values of the *t*-statistic.

The *t*-statistics calculated for *t*-tests performed on samples that are assumed to have equal and unequal variances are shown in Table 24.6.

Table 24.4 DTS data for two samples with unequal variances.

	Material A	Material B
	18.0	22.0
	20.0	24.5
	25.0	25.0
	30.0	25.9
	30.7	26.0
	33.0	26.2
	35.0	27.0
	38.5	27.3
	41.2	28.0
	45.3	33.0
Mean	31.7	26.5
S.Dev.	8.9	2.8
Variance	78.6	8.1
CofV, %	28.0	10.7

It can be seen from this table that whereas the t-statistics were the same for the data under both assumptions, the values of t_c (and their corresponding probabilities) differ for calculations based on the two assumptions. The t-statistic for data with unequal variances has a higher t_c, and a lower probability, than that for equal variances.

COMPARISON OF TWO MEANS FOR PAIRED SAMPLES

In two-sample testing, it is assumed that the two samples are independent and any one particular datum item in one sample has no association

Table 24.5 F-ratio test for data in Table 22.4.

	Material A	Material B
Mean	31.67	26.49
Variance	78.60	8.07
Observations	10	10
df	9	9
F	9.75	
$P(F \leq f)$ one-tailed	0.00115	
$F_{critical}$ one-tailed	3.18	

Table 24.6 Calculated values of the *t*-statistic for data in Table 22.4 when unequal and equal variances are assumed.

	Unequal variances		Equal variances	
	Material A	**Material B**	**Material A**	**Material B**
Mean	31.67	26.49	31.67	26.49
Variance	78.60	8.07	78.60	8.07
Observations	10	10	10	10
Pooled variance			43.33	
Hypothesized mean difference	0		0	
df	11		18	
t-statistic	1.760		1.760	
$P(T \leq t)$ one-tailed	0.053		0.048	
$t_{critical}$ one-tailed	1.796		1.734	
$P(T \leq t)$ two-tailed	0.106		0.095	
$t_{critical}$ two-tailed	2.201		2.101	

with any specific datum in the other sample. There are, however, situations in which each observation in Group A correlates with an observation in Group B. An example of this might be when pairs of specimens are prepared under the same conditions and one specimen is placed into Group A and the other into Group B, with each pair being identified. If, for

Table 24.7 Strengths (MPa) of matched pairs of specimens exposed to water and dilute alkali solution for 1 week.

	Water	**Alkali**
	20.0	17.6
	21.2	18.3
	22.3	19.2
	25.7	23.4
	28.4	26.7
	30.3	27.4
	31.0	28.6
	31.9	29.9
	33.5	30.1
	34.7	30.8
Mean	27.9	25.2
S.Dev.	5.3	5.2
Variance	28.1	26.7
CofV, %	19.0	20.5

Table 24.8   Results from a paired-sample *t*-test.

	Water	Alkali
Mean	27.9	25.2
Variance	28.1	26.7
Observations	10	10
Pearson correlation	0.992	
Hypothesized mean difference	0	
df	9	
t-statistic	12.807	
$P(T \leq t)$ one-tailed	0.000	
$t_{critical}$ one-tailed	1.833	
$P(T \leq t)$ two-tailed	0.000	
$t_{critical}$ two-tailed	2.262	

example, ten pairs of glass ionomer cement specimens are prepared and the Group A specimens are immersed in distilled water for 1 week whereas the specimens in Group B are immersed in dilute alkali solution, comparison of the two groups will determine if the alkali bath had a detrimental effect on the dental cement.

The measured strengths for the paired specimens in the two groups of matched samples are shown in Table 24.7.

Excel will perform a *t*-test for matched pairs (under *data analysis*: *t*-test: *paired two-sample for means*), as shown in Table 24.8.

Comparing the calculated *t*-statistic with the critical *t* values for one-tailed and two-tailed tests clearly shows that there is a statistically significant difference between the two sets of data ($P = 0.000$).

Note that Table 24.8 contains a parameter known as the Pearson correlation coefficient (r) and this number measures the degree of association between two variables. A positive value indicates that as the values in Group A increase, those in Group B will also increase. Conversely, a negative correlation indicates that as values in Group A increase, those in Group B decrease. Thus, the correlation coefficient measures the strength of a linear relationship between two variables and the correlation between the two variables improves as r approaches unity ($r \rightarrow 1.0$).

Analysis of Variance

One of the most useful techniques in statistics is *analysis of variance* (*ANOVA*), a method of comparing the means of two or more populations. Previous chapters discussed the standard deviation as a measure of the dispersion of values about their mean as well as the relationship of the standard deviation (and variance) to the standard error of the mean. Also discussed was the use of these values to test whether or not the difference between two sets of data was statistically significant.

Data analysis becomes more complex when several sets of observations are to be compared. Although it is possible to perform a series of *t* tests in which each pair of data sets is compared in turn, this would be very time-consuming and this approach may be invalid because of the escalating risk of Type I errors with an increasing number of *t* tests.

This situation can be avoided by using the very useful technique of ANOVA. Normally, calculating all the various parameters required for an ANOVA test is tedious but Excel incorporates the subroutine to perform different types of ANOVA procedures.

COMPARISON OF TWO SAMPLES

The Excel spreadsheet will calculate a number of statistics from the entered data and then calculate the value of the *F statistic*, the critical value of *F* for significance (F_{crit}), and the probability associated with the calculated *F value*. This is demonstrated using as an example the DTS values previously shown in Table 24.1, shown here as Table 25.1.

To perform an ANOVA on these data, in Excel under the drop-down menu of *tools*: *data analysis* click on *ANOVA: single factor* and follow the prompts. A single-factor analysis, also known as a *one-way analysis*, is performed since only one factor is being tested, namely the effect of the type of material on diametral tensile strength.

Table 25.1 Diametral strengths (MPa) of two restorative materials.

Material A	Material B
20.0	22.0
28.5	24.5
29.0	25.0
30.0	25.9
30.7	26.0
30.8	26.2
31.0	27.0
32.0	27.3
33.0	28.0
42.0	33.0

The table of statistics (Table 25.2) will be calculated by Excel. The provided data under SUMMARY are:

1. *Count*: the number of samples in each group (N)
2. *Sum*: the sum of the values in each group
3. *Average*: the mean value for each group
4. *Variance*: the variance of the data in each group (where variance is the square of the standard deviation)

Table 25.2 Calculated statistics using the Excel spreadsheet for data in Table 25.1.

ANOVA: single factor						
SUMMARY						
Groups	**Count**	**Sum**	**Average**	**Variance**		
Material A	10	307	30.7	28.6		
Material B	10	264.9	26.5	8.1		
ANOVA						
Source of variation	**SS**	**df**	**MS**	**F**	**P value**	**F_crit**
Between groups	88.62	1	88.62	4.83	0.04	4.41
Within groups	330.07	18	18.34			
Total	418.69	19				

Under ANOVA, the spreadsheet provides additional items of statistical information using the different headings:

a. *Source of variation*: When testing data, there are two sources of variation, the variation between the two groups and the variation with each group.
b. *SS (sum of squares)—between groups*: This is the sum of the squares of the deviation of each datum item from the mean of *all* specimens in the two sets of data. This calculation indicates the effects arising between the two test groups.

   SS (sum of squares)—within groups: This is the sum of the squares of the deviation of each datum item *in* a group from the mean of that group. This calculation indicates the effects arising from within each test group.
c. *df (degrees of freedom)—between groups*: There are two groups, therefore $df = 1$.

   df (degrees of freedom)—within groups: There are ten specimens in group, therefore the degrees of freedom $df = (N_A - 1) + (N_B - 1) = (10 - 1) + (10 - 1) = 18$.
d. *MS (Mean sum of squares)—between groups*: This is the estimate of the between groups variance and is given by $SS_{between}/df = 88.62/1 = 88.62$

   MS (Mean sum of squares)—within groups: This is the estimate of the within groups variance and is given by $SS_{within}/df = 330.07/18 = 18.34$.
e. *F*: The variance ratio, $F = \dfrac{\text{between sample variance estimate}}{\text{within sample variance estimate}} = \dfrac{88.62}{18.34} = 4.83$.
f. *P value*: Probability of significance of the variance ratio.
g. F_{crit}: The critical value of F for significance.

Since the value of F in the *variance ratio test* (or *Snedecor's F test*) is greater than F_{crit}, it can be concluded that there is a statistically significant difference between the two data groups. The significance of the difference is 0.04% or $P = 0.04$, that is, $P < 0.05$.

MULTIPLE SAMPLE COMPARISONS

The F test is very useful when data sets comprising more than two groups are to be tested. Table 25.3 shows an example of four groups of five children taken at random from four locales. Three locales have fluoridated water supplies whereas one locale (Group 3 children) is fluoride-free. Is

Table 25.3 DMF scores for four groups of children.

A	B	C	D
2	3	6	4
3	4	8	3
2	3	7	3
3	4	4	4
1	2	5	2

there a difference in the DMF (decayed, missing or filled teeth) scores for the four groups of children?

Since only one factor is being tested, that is, whether the presence of fluoride in drinking water reduces dental decay as reflected by the DMF score, a *single factor* or *one-way ANOVA* is performed.

The analysis is performed in Excel following the same procedure as above, and the tabulated results of the calculations are shown in Table 25.4.

The calculated F score (11.64) is markedly higher than F_{crit} (3.239), clearly indicating a statistically significant difference among the four

Table 25.4 One-way ANOVA of the DMF scores for four groups of children.

ANOVA: single factor						

SUMMARY

Groups	Count	Sum	Average	Variance		
A	5	11	2.2	0.7		
B	5	16	3.2	0.7		
C	5	30	6	2.5		
D	5	16	3.2	0.7		

ANOVA

Source of variation	SS	df	MS	F	P value	F_{crit}
Between groups	40.15	3	13.38	11.64	0.0003	3.2389
Within groups	18.4	16	1.15			
Total	58.55	19				

groups of DMF scores. The probability of significance is $P = 0.0003$, and it can be concluded that the difference is *highly significant* since $P \leq 0.001$.

While ANOVA has shown that there is a difference among the four sets of data, identifying the source of that difference involves multiple comparisons. This will be discussed in Chapter 27.

TWO-WAY ANOVA

In many studies, the researcher may want to investigate two or more factors simultaneously. While it is efficient to run all the samples in a strength test study at the same time, distinguishing between the various data sets (the strength results) requires a more complex analysis. This analysis is known as a *two-factor* or *two-way* ANOVA and, fortunately, this analysis can also be performed in Excel.

An example might be determining the strengths of three composite restorative materials when cured with a standard visible light unit, a high-intensity light, and a laser energy source with four specimens ($N = 4$) tested for each material and each curing method (Table 25.5). This is an example of a two-way ANOVA since two factors, the composite material and the curing system, are under investigation.

To perform an ANOVA on these data in Excel under *tools: data analysis* click on *ANOVA: two-factor with replication* and follow the prompts. Because four specimens were fabricated independently from each material

Table 25.5 Strengths of three restorative materials polymerized with three curing lights with four specimens tested of each material and each curing light.

	Material A	Material B	Material C
Standard	12.7	12.9	13.9
Standard	13.3	14.2	14.5
Standard	12.8	13.7	13.7
Standard	11.9	13.4	14.1
High intensity	13.9	13.7	15.7
High intensity	14.1	15.1	16.4
High intensity	14.3	14.9	16.9
High intensity	13.1	15.2	15.3
Laser	15.3	15.8	17.5
Laser	16.2	16.3	18.9
Laser	14.9	16.5	17.8
Laser	16.4	15.7	18.3

Table 25.6 Two-way ANOVA with replication of the strengths of restorative materials.

ANOVA: two-factor with replication

SUMMARY

Standard	Material A	Material B	Material C	Total
Count	4	4	4	12
Sum	50.7	54.2	56.2	161.1
Average	12.68	13.55	14.05	13.43
Variance	0.34	0.30	0.12	0.56
High intensity				
Count	4	4	4	12
Sum	55.4	58.9	64.3	178.6
Average	13.85	14.73	16.08	14.88
Variance	0.28	0.48	0.51	1.26
Laser				
Count	4	4	4	12
Sum	62.8	64.3	72.5	199.6
Average	15.70	16.08	18.13	16.63
Variance	0.51	0.15	0.38	1.52
Total				
Count	12	12	12	
Sum	168.9	177.4	193	
Average	14.08	14.78	16.08	
Variance	2.00	1.41	3.29	

ANOVA

Source of variation	SS	df	MS	F	P value	F_{crit}
Sample	61.93	2	30.965	91.199	0.000	3.354
Columns	24.90	2	12.450	36.668	0.000	3.354
Interaction	2.66	4	0.664	1.957	0.130	2.728
Within	9.17	27	0.340			
Total	98.66	35				

and using each curing method, every sample is independent and the data are said to be *replicated*. The results of the Excel ANOVA calculations are shown in Table 25.6.

Table 25.6 contains a term, *interaction*, not found with one-way ANOVA. Generally, in a study testing the effects of two factors X and Y,

Table 25.7 Strengths of three restorative materials polymerized with three curing lights.

	Material A	Material B	Material C
Standard	12.7	12.9	13.9
Standard	13.3	14.2	14.5
Standard	12.8	13.7	13.7
Standard	11.9	13.4	14.1
High intensity	13.9	13.7	15.7
High intensity	14.1	15.1	16.4
High intensity	14.3	14.9	16.9
High intensity	13.1	15.2	15.3
Laser	15.3	15.8	19.7
Laser	16.2	16.3	20.1
Laser	14.9	16.5	21.3
Laser	16.4	15.7	20.5

the variability between Group X data and Group Y data is not equal to the sum of the sums of squares. The difference not taken into account is the *interaction* between factors X and Y, designated as the $X \times Y$ interaction. The statistic *within source of variation* represents differences arising from normal sampling variations.

This is illustrated in Table 25.7, which shows a hypothetical example of interactive effects in evaluating the strengths of restorative materials. One material (Material C) contains a catalyst specifically designed for use with laser curing lights and is claimed to yield a higher degree of polymerization during curing. The use of this catalyst should result in a measurably greater strength of the final polymerized material.

The Excel-generated statistics using a *two-way ANOVA with replication* analysis (Table 25.8) shows that there is a statistically significant interactive effect within the data sets.

Based on this analysis, it could be deduced that the catalyst for laser light curing has a beneficial effect on the strength of Material C.

REPLICATION

The term *replication* was mentioned above. Replicated data comprise measurements made on specimens independent of each other. In other words, if the data comprise N samples, then one and only one measurement was made on each individual specimen within a population of N specimens. Making several measurements on the same specimen is *pseudoreplication*

Table 25.8 Two-way ANOVA with replication of the strengths of restorative materials.

ANOVA: two-factor with replication

SUMMARY

Standard	Material A	Material B	Material C	Total
Count	4	4	4	12
Sum	50.7	54.2	56.2	161.1
Average	12.675	13.55	14.05	13.425
Variance	0.336	0.297	0.117	0.557
High intensity				
Count	4	4	4	12
Sum	55.4	58.9	64.3	178.6
Average	13.85	14.73	16.08	14.88
Variance	0.277	0.483	0.509	1.260
Laser				
Count	4	4	4	12
Sum	62.8	64.3	81.6	208.7
Average	15.7	16.08	20.40	17.39
Variance	0.513	0.149	0.467	5.270
Total				
Count	12	12	12	
Sum	168.9	177.4	202.1	
Average	14.1	14.8	16.8	
Variance	2.0	1.4	7.9	

ANOVA

Source of variation	SS	df	MS	F	P value	F_{crit}
Sample	96.61	2	48.306	138.163	0.000	3.354
Columns	49.57	2	24.786	70.892	0.000	3.354
Interaction	18.94	4	4.734	13.541	0.000	2.728
Within	9.44	27	0.350			
Total	174.56	35				

and is invalid. The exception to this rule, of course, is when the same parameter is measured over a period of time in order to evaluate a time-based change in that parameter. Examples of such time-based series might be measurements of blood pressure or glucose levels in human patients over an extended period of time, etc.

Table 25.9 Strengths of three restorative materials polymerized with three curing lights tested without replication.

	Material A	Material B	Material C
Standard	12.1	11.9	11.8
High intensity	13.3	12.7	13.7
Laser	14.3	13.8	15.4

It is possible to perform a multisample ANOVA with only one sample in each cell, that is, a *two-way ANOVA without replication* with only one specimen being tested of each material and each curing method. An example of the data obtained in this type of study is shown in Table 25.9.

Calculating the means and their standard deviations of the columns (the materials) and the rows (curing methods) (Table 25.10) suggests that there are no differences among materials (i.e., among the columns) but there might be differences among the rows (i.e., among the curing methods).

To determine whether these differences are statistically significant, an ANOVA can be performed. The procedure in Excel is to click on *ANOVA: two-factor without replication* under *tools: data analysis* and follow the prompts. The calculated statistics are shown in Table 25.11.

The tabulated statistics indicate that there is no statistically significant ($P = 0.202$) difference among the columns, that is, among the three materials. However, there does appear to be a statistically significant difference ($P = 0.006$) among the rows of data, that is, among the curing methods.

The *error factor* in Table 25.11 is the residual or within-treatment sum of squares and represents differences due to normal sampling variations.

The data in Tables 25.10 and 25.11 suggest that whereas differences may not exist among the three materials, the three different light sources do

Table 25.10 Means and standard deviations for data in Table 25.9.

		Material A	Material B	Material C	Columns		
					Mean	S.Dev.	CofV, %
	Standard	12.1	11.9	11.8	11.9	0.2	1.3
	High intensity	13.3	12.7	13.7	13.2	0.5	3.8
	Laser	14.3	13.8	15.4	14.5	0.8	5.6
Rows	Mean	13.2	12.8	13.6			
	S.Dev.	1.1	1.0	1.8			
	CofV, %	8.3	7.5	13.2			

Table 25.11 A two-factor ANOVA without replication.

ANOVA: two-factor without replication

SUMMARY

	Count	Sum	Average	Variance
Standard	3	35.8	11.9	0.0
High intensity	3	39.7	13.2	0.3
Laser	3	43.5	14.5	0.7
Material A	3	39.7	13.2	1.2
Material B	3	38.4	12.8	0.9
Material C	3	40.9	13.6	3.2

ANOVA

Source of variation	SS	df	MS	F	P value	F_{crit}
Rows	9.88	2	4.941	23.222	0.006	6.944
Columns	1.04	2	0.521	2.449	0.202	6.944
Error	0.85	4	0.213			
Total	11.78	8				

affect strength. The conclusion that could be drawn here is that the study findings suggest that the curing method affects strength but probably not the material. The sensible researcher should then repeat the study but with a greater number of specimens to increase the *power* of the ANOVA. Power in statistical analysis is discussed in Chapter 26.

MULTIVARIATE ANALYSIS

ANOVA is a very powerful tool in statistical analysis and can be used to analyze for statistical significance in sets of data with numerous columns (e.g., different types of materials) and many rows (e.g., different treatment methods). If only two factors affect the data, then Excel may be used for the statistical analysis.

When a study involves multiple factors that affect the data, then the analysis involved is beyond both the scope of this book and the built-in subroutines of Excel. In such cases, specialty statistical software or a statistician should be involved in the data analysis.

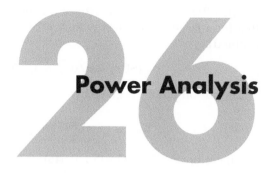

Power Analysis

In virtually every statistical analysis, the greater the number of samples being tested, the more accurate is the analysis. Increasing the number of samples is said to increase the *power* of the test. In fact, statistical consultants to editorial boards of many scientific and biomedical journals require authors submitting manuscripts to specify the power of the statistical testing they performed.

TYPE I AND TYPE II ERRORS

The probability of a *Type I error* is the likelihood of rejecting a true null hypothesis (see Chapter 23), and is equal to the *a priori* significance level of the hypothesis test (α). A test performed at the 5% significance level has a probability of a Type I error of $\alpha = 0.05$, that is, there is only a 5% chance of rejecting H_0 as false when in fact H_0 is true. The probability of a *Type II error* (the probability of not rejecting a false null hypothesis) is denoted by β.

A hypothetical example is as follows: a new glass ionomer cement (GIC) is claimed by the manufacturer to have a mean elastic modulus of 25 GPa with a standard deviation of 3 GPa; that is, $\mu = 25$ GPa and $\sigma = 3$ GPa. The manufacturer is claiming that the new glass ionomer has a markedly greater elastic modulus than that of a traditional GIC, namely 20 GPa.

The null hypothesis (the manufacturer's claim) H_0: $\mu = 25$ GPa; the alternative hypothesis, put forward by an independent testing laboratory, is that the mean elastic modulus is less than 25 GPa, or H_1: $\mu < 25$ GPa.

A decision has to be made regarding the cut-off value of the modulus (c) at which the null hypothesis is rejected. If a significance level of 0.05 is adopted, the value of c can be calculated using the z-score (z-statistic) for this significance level, namely $z_{\text{cut-off}} = -1.645$ (the value of z for which 5% of the area under the normal curve lies in the left-hand tail; see

Chapter 21). The standard error of the mean (SE $\bar{x}$) is given by $\sigma/\sqrt{N}$, so that for a large sample test with $N = 30$ (i.e., the data are normally distributed):

$$(SE_{\bar{x}}) = \sigma/\sqrt{N} = 3/\sqrt{30} = 0.548$$

The cut-off point c is given by:

$$z_{cut-off} = -1.645 = \frac{c - 25}{SE_{\bar{x}}} = \frac{c - 25}{0.548}$$

and therefore $c = 25 - (1.645 \times 0.548) = 25 - 0.90 = 24.1$ GPa.

Thus, at a 5% significance level, if the mean elastic modulus ($\bar{x}$) measured by the independent laboratory is less than 24.1 GPa ($\bar{x} < 24.1$), H_0 can be rejected in favor of H_1.

In this case, a Type I error (rejection of a true null hypothesis) would be *to reject* the manufacturer's claimed modulus of 25 GPa when in fact the mean modulus actually is 25 GPa. A Type II error (not rejecting a false null hypothesis) would be *not* to reject the manufacturer's claim (mean modulus = 25 GPa) when in fact the mean modulus is less than 25 GPa.

A Type I error would result in bad publicity for the manufacturer and potentially could lead to law suits being filed because, in effect, the independent laboratory is suggesting that the manufacturer had made a false claim. A Type II error would prevent the independent laboratory from rejecting the manufacturer's claim when in reality, the claim is false. This might not upset the manufacturer but would be misleading to the consumer (the dentist using the new product).

The probability of making a Type I error is 0.05, that is, the significance level (α). In the present example, H_0 is true and not rejected if $\bar{x} \geq 24.1$ at a 5% significance level. The probability of making a Type II error is β, and depends upon the sample size and the significance level (α). This probability can be calculated because it is the area of the tail to the right of $z_{cut-off}$.

If the true mean elastic modulus (μ) is 24.5 GPa, the z-score of the measured modulus 24.1 is:

$$z = \frac{24.1 - 24.5}{0.548} = -0.730.$$

The probability of a Type II error β is given by the sum of the area in the tail to the right of $z = -0.730$ (0.267 from tabulated areas under the standard normal curve) and the area under the normal curve from $\bar{x}$ (the mean value) to the limit of the right-hand side of the curve $z = 4.0$ (0.500) (Figure 26.1).

The total area is $0.500 + 0.267 = 0.767$. Thus, the probability of making a Type II error is 0.767; that is, there is a 77% chance that the independent

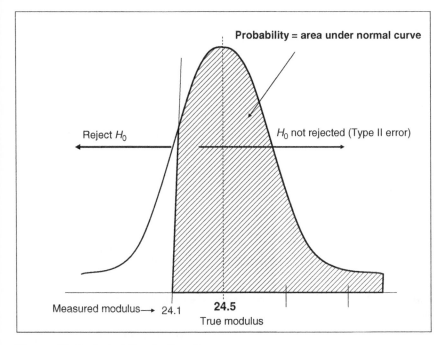

Figure 26.1   Probability of a Type II error.

laboratory will not reject the manufacturer's claim of an elastic modulus of 25 GPa even though $\mu = 24.5$ GPa.

If the number of samples is increased to 60 ($N = 60$), the standard error of the mean $(SE_{\bar{x}}) = \sigma/\sqrt{N} = 3/\sqrt{60} = 0.387$

The cut-off point c is given by:

$$z_{\text{cut-off}} = -1.645 = \frac{c - 25}{SE_{\bar{x}}} = \frac{c - 25}{0.387}$$

and therefore $c = 25 - (1.645 \times 0.387) = 25 - 0.637 = 24.36$ GPa.

If the true mean elastic modulus is 24.5 GPa, the z-score of the measured modulus 24.36 is:

$$z = \frac{24.36 - 24.5}{0.387} = -0.362$$

and the probability of a Type II error is given by the sum of the area in the tail to the right of $z = -0.362$ and that of the area from $z = 0$ to $z = 4.0$ (Figure 26.1). The area for $z = -0.362$ to $z = 0$ is 0.141 from a table of areas under the standard normal curve so that the total area of the indi-cated region is $0.500 + 0.141 = 0.641$. Thus, the probability of a Type II error is about 64%, indicating that increasing the sample size from 30 to

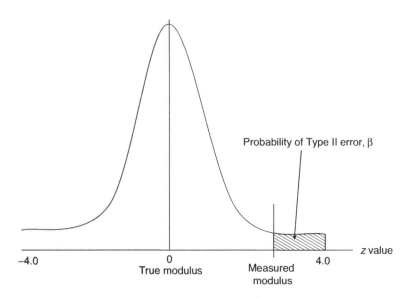

Figure 26.2 Probability of a Type II error when sample mean is greater than true mean.

60 decreases the probability of a Type II error (as well as that of a Type I error).

In the event that the true elastic modulus is 23 GPa, the z-score for a modulus of 24.1 determined by the independent laboratory is:

$$z = \frac{24.1 - 23}{0.548} = 2.01$$

and the probability of a Type II error is given by the area under the tail (Figure 26.2).

The area of the tail is given by the difference between the total area under the right side of the curve (0.500) and the area from $z = 0$ to $z = 2.01$ (0.478 from tables).

The area of tail (probability of Type II error, β) = $0.500 - 0.478 = 0.022$ so that the probability of a Type II error, $\beta = 0.022$ or 2.2%.

It should be noted, however, that in the "real world," it is highly unlikely that the independent laboratory would actually detect such a small difference in the elastic modulus even without increasing the sample size.

POWER IN STATISTICAL TESTING

The *power* of a statistical test is defined as $1 - \beta$, where β is the probability of committing a Type II error. Thus, the power of a statistical test is the probability that the test will correctly reject the null hypothesis (H_0) when it is false.

In the example worked above, when the sample size was increased from 30 to 60, β decreased from 0.767 to 0.641 (from 76 to 64%) and the power $(1 - \beta)$ increased from 0.233 to 0.359 (23–36%). Similarly, when the true mean of the elastic modulus of the new GIC was 23 GPa, the value of β dropped to 0.022 (2.2%) and the power correspondingly increased to 0.978 (98%). Analogous to the effect of sample size, it can be shown that as the significance level α increases, the power of a test will decrease.

ESTIMATING THE POWER OF A *t*-TEST

It is possible to calculate the probability of detecting a true difference between a measured mean and a claimed mean. Table 26.1 indicates the findings of a strength test on a dental material for which the manufacturer claims a mean strength of 32 MPa. The question to be asked is: what is the probability of detecting a true difference of at least 2 MPa between tested samples and the manufacturer's claim?

The sample size $N = 10$ and therefore $df = 9$, and the variance of the data is 4.5. If it is required to know the probability of correctly rejecting a

Table 26.1 Strength data for a dental material (in MPa).

	29.4
	29.9
	30.1
	30.6
	30.7
	30.9
	31.5
	31.9
	32.7
	33.3
	34.1
	36.8
Mean	31.8
S.Dev.	2.1
Variance	4.5

false H_0, the power of the t-test must be estimated:

$$t_{\beta(1),df} = \frac{\delta}{\sqrt{(s^2/N)}} - t_{\alpha,df}$$

where δ is the difference between μ (30 MPa) and the sample $\bar{x}$ (31.8 MPa) that is to be measured, $t_{\alpha(2),df}$ is the t statistic for the significance level α and the df in a two-tailed test (the value of this statistic drawn for a table of t values is 2.262) and $t_{\beta(1),df}$ is the t value of β at $df = 9$.

$$t_{\beta(1),df} = \frac{2.0}{\sqrt{(4.5/10)}} - 2.262 = 0.719$$

Tabulated t values indicate that for $df = 9$, $\beta > 0.20$ and therefore the power is: $1 - \beta < 0.80$.

If $t = 0.719$ is considered to be a normal deviate, $\beta = 0.24$ (from tables) and a more exact estimate of the power is obtained, namely 0.76 (76%).

A comparable calculation can be used to estimate the required sample size (N) to detect a difference of 2.0 MPa. Using the same data in Table 26.1, if $\alpha = 0.05$ with a 90% probability of detecting $\delta = 2.0$ and rearranging the equation:

$$N = \frac{s^2}{\delta^2} - \left(t_{\alpha(2),df} + t_{\beta(1),df}\right)^2$$

From tables, $t_{\alpha(2),df} = 2.262$, $t_{\beta(1),df} = 1.383$ whereas $s^2 = 4.5$, $\delta = 2.0$, and $df = 9$ (for $N = 10$), so that:

$$N = \frac{4.5}{(2.0)^2} \times (2.262 + 1.383)^2 = 14.95$$

and it can be concluded that a minimum sample size of 15 is required.

It follows from this that for any proposed statistical testing method, the power of the test and the value of α will decide the appropriate sample size (the value of N) for the study. It is possible to calculate the power and required sample size for ANOVA testing but these calculations involve the χ^2 (chi-square) statistic, a subject discussed in Chapter 28.

Performing any of the above calculations manually is tedious but computer programs now are available to perform this task. Readers interested in further discussion of this subject can consult the monographs suggested in the Appendix.

Multiple Comparisons

During the discussion of the analysis of variance, Chapter 25, it was stated that even though ANOVA could indicate that differences exist among data, identifying the source of those differences required additional testing, the subject of this chapter. Many *multiple comparisons* tests have been developed to analyze the reasons that made ANOVA reject the null hypothesis. These tests are known as *post hoc* or *a posteriori* tests.

Unfortunately, Excel does not have the capability of performing multiple comparison testing and other software must be used. For convenience, the approach to multiple comparisons will be based upon the ProStat program (Poly Software International, Pearl River, NY).

When performing a multiple comparison using ProStat, the data from Table 25.7 (shown below as Table 27.1) have to be rearranged (Table 27.2) and a task can easily be performed in Excel by cutting and pasting.

These data can then be copied and dropped into ProStat and the column headings inserted into the ProStat spreadsheet (Figure 27.1).

Under the drop-down menu, the user is presented with several choices (Figure 27.2).

The column of data to be tested must be highlighted and then the appropriate analytical test is selected. Selection of a multiple comparison test is discussed below. In this case, the Scheffé test was used (Figure 27.3).

After *OK* is pressed, ProStat performs the analysis and a multiple comparison report is produced (Figure 27.4).

The report shown in Figure 27.4 contains a lot of information and the data provided in each block are the following:

a. *Selected data columns*: It indicates the columns analyzed and gives the means, variances, and standard deviations of each column.
b. *One-way ANOVA*: One-way ANOVA indicating a statistically significant between the columns.

Table 27.1 Strengths of three restorative materials polymerized with three curing lights with four specimens tested of each material and each curing light.

	Material A	**Material B**	**Material C**
Standard	12.7	12.9	13.9
Standard	13.3	14.2	14.5
Standard	12.8	13.7	13.7
Standard	11.9	13.4	14.1
High intensity	13.9	13.7	15.7
High intensity	14.1	15.1	16.4
High intensity	14.3	14.9	16.9
High intensity	13.1	15.2	15.3
Laser	15.3	15.8	19.7
Laser	16.2	16.3	20.1
Laser	14.9	16.5	21.3
Laser	16.4	15.7	20.5

c. *Scheffé's method*: This block places the column means in ascending order and provides a matrix showing the arithmetic differences between the column means.

d. *Rejection matrix*: This block indicates the comparisons for which H_0 is rejected (i.e., there is a statistically significant difference between columns); for example, there is a statistically significant difference between Material B—high-intensity light cured and Material A—standard light cured.

e. *Probability matrix*: This block shows the probability of the observed difference having occurred by chance, for example, in the case of Material B—high-intensity light cured and Material A—standard light cured, the probability is 0.015.

f. *Critical range matrix*: This block shows the critical range of the difference between means at a 95% confidence level.

Table 27.2 Reorganized data from Table 27.1.

Material A			**Material B**			**Material C**		
Standard	High intensity	Laser	Standard	High intensity	Laser	Standard	High intensity	Laser
12.7	13.9	15.3	12.9	13.7	15.8	13.9	15.7	19.7
13.3	14.1	16.2	14.2	15.1	16.3	14.5	16.4	20.1
12.8	14.3	14.9	13.7	14.9	16.5	13.7	16.9	21.3
11.9	13.1	16.4	13.4	15.2	15.7	14.1	15.3	20.5

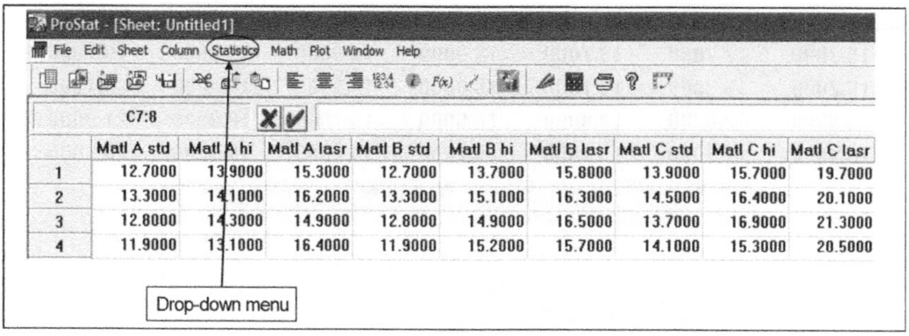

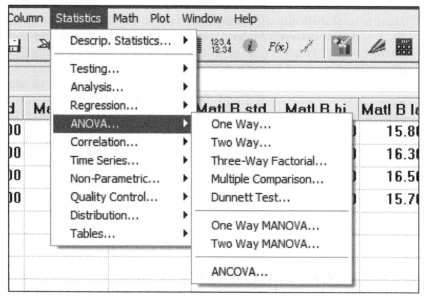

Figure 27.1 Data from Table 27.2 placed in ProStat spreadsheet (drop-down menu indicated with an arrow).

Finally, the report shows the results of Bartlett's chi-square (χ^2) analysis of the homogeneity of variance and the probability of that difference occurring by chance. The χ^2 test is discussed in Chapter 28.

Perusal of the data and Scheffé report permits a number of conclusions to be drawn. These include:

1. There is no statistically significant difference in the strengths of Materials A, B, and C when cured with the standard light.

Figure 27.2 Drop-down menu in ProStat spreadsheet for multiple comparisons.

Matl A lasr	Matl B std	Matl B hi	Matl B lasr	Matl C std	Matl C hi	Matl C lasr
15.3000	12.7000	13.7000	15.8000	13.9000	15.7000	19.7000
16.2000	13.3000	15.1000	16.3000	14.5000	16.4000	20.1000
14.9000	12.8000	14.9000	16.5000	13.7000	16.9000	21.3000
16.4000	11.9000	15.2000	15.7000	14.1000	15.3000	20.5000

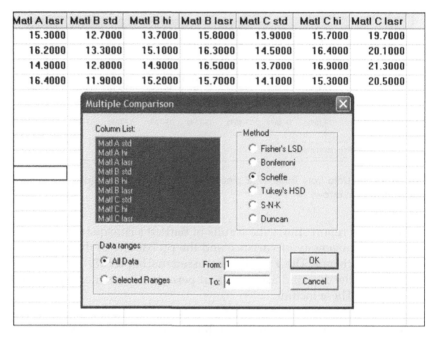

Figure 27.3 Highlighting data columns to be tested and selecting the analytical method in ProStat.

2. There is no statistically significant difference in the strengths of Materials A and B or between Materials B and C when cured with the high intensity light. However, there is a statistically significant difference ($P = 0.006$) between Materials A and C.
3. There is no statistically significant difference in the strengths of Materials A and B when cured with the laser light, but laser light cured Material C is stronger ($P = 0.000$) than laser-cured Materials A and B.

Obviously, many more comparisons can be made based on the multiple comparison report, for example, standard light versus high-intensity strengths for each material, strengths comparing material types for each light source, etc. The analysis elucidates the ANOVA findings in Table 25.8 and clearly demonstrates that the new laser-sensitive catalyst in Material C has the intended effect.

MULTIPLE COMPARISON TESTS

The drop-down menu in Figure 27.3 and most statistics textbooks indicate that there are a number of multiple comparison tests (Table 27.3), each

```
=========================================================
        Multiple comparison report
        Data file name: Composite material strengths
=========================================================
Selected data columns:
Matl A-std: Mean = 12.675000, Variance = 0.335833, StdDev = 0.579511
MatlA-hi: Mean = 13.850000, Variance = 0.276667, StdDev = 0.525991
MatlA-lasr: Mean = 15.700000, Variance = 0.513333, StdDev = 0.716473
MatlB-std: Mean = 13.550000, Variance = 0.296667, StdDev = 0.544671
MatlB-hi: Mean = 14.725000, Variance = 0.482500, StdDev = 0.694622
MatlB-lasr: Mean = 16.075000, Variance = 0.149167, StdDev = 0.386221
MatlC-std: Mean = 14.050000, Variance = 0.116667, StdDev = 0.341565
MatlC-hi: Mean = 16.075000, Variance = 0.509167, StdDev = 0.713559
MatlC-lasr: Mean = 20.400000, Variance = 0.466667, StdDev = 0.683130
=========================================================

One-way ANOVA
```

Source	df	SumofSq	MeanofSq	F value	P value
Between groups	8	165.1200	20.6400	59.0339	0.0000
Within groups	27	9.4400	0.3496		

Total	35	174.5600			

```
Scheffe's method:
Mean values:
Matl A-std     12.67500
MatlB-std      13.55000
MatlA-hi       13.85000
MatlC-std      14.05000
MatlB-hi       14.72500
MatlA-lasr     15.70000
MatlB-lasr     16.07500
MatlC-hi       16.07500
MatlC-lasr     20.40000
```

Mean difference matrix:

	Matl A-std	MatlB-std	MatlA-hi	MatlC-std	MatlB-hi	MatlA-lasr	MatlB-lasr	MatlC-hi
MatlB-std	0.875							
MatlA-hi	1.175	0.300						
MatlC-std	1.375	0.500	0.200					
MatlB-hi	2.050	1.175	0.875	0.675				
MatlA-lasr	3.025	2.150	1.850	1.650	0.975			
MatlB-lasr	3.400	2.525	2.225	2.025	1.350	0.375		
MatlC-hi	3.400	2.525	2.225	2.025	1.350	0.375	0.000	
MatlC-lasr	7.725	6.850	6.550	6.350	5.675	4.700	4.325	4.325

Rejection matrix:

	Matl A-std	MatlB-std	MatlA-hi	MatlC-std	MatlB-hi	MatlA-lasr	MatlB-lasr	MatlC-hi
MatlB-std	No							
MatlA-hi	No	No						
MatlC-std	No	No	No					
MatlB-hi	Yes	No	No	No				
MatlA-lasr	Yes	Yes	Yes	No	No			
MatlB-lasr	Yes	Yes	Yes	Yes	No	No		
MatlC-hi	Yes	Yes	Yes	Yes	No	No	No	
MatlC-lasr	Yes	Yes	Yes	Yes	Yes	Yes	Yes	Yes

Figure 27.4 Multiple comparison report generated by ProStat for the data in Table 27.2.

```
Probability matrix:
        Matl A-std MatlB-std  MatlA-hi MatlC-std  MatlB-hiMatlA-lasrMatlB-lasr  MatlC-hi
MatlB-std    0.810
MatlA-hi     0.467   1.000
MatlC-std    0.262   0.992    1.000
MatlB-hi     0.015   0.467    0.810    0.949
MatlA-lasr   0.000   0.009    0.039    0.094    0.705
MatlB-lasr   0.000   0.001    0.006    0.017    0.284    0.999
MatlC-hi     0.000   0.001    0.006    0.017    0.284    0.999    1.000
MatlC-lasr   0.000   0.000    0.000    0.000    0.000    0.000    0.000    0.000

Critical range matrix (95% confidence):
        Matl A-std MatlB-std  MatlA-hi MatlC-std  MatlB-hiMatlA-lasrMatlB-lasr  MatlC-hi
MatlB-std    1.796
MatlA-hi     1.796   1.796
MatlC-std    1.796   1.796    1.796
MatlB-hi     1.796   1.796    1.796    1.796
MatlA-lasr   1.796   1.796    1.796    1.796    1.796
MatlB-lasr   1.796   1.796    1.796    1.796    1.796    1.796
MatlC-hi     1.796   1.796    1.796    1.796    1.796    1.796    1.796
MatlC-lasr   1.796   1.796    1.796    1.796    1.796    1.796    1.796    1.796

Test of homogeneity of variance:
    Bartlett's chi-square:        2.71612549
    Degree of freedom:            8
    Probability:                  0.95089068
=================================================================
```

Figure 27.4 (*Continued*)

developed for a different purpose and analytical capability. The aim of any multiple comparison test is to retain the same overall rate of false positives and, as a result, the standards for each comparison must be more stringent. Reducing the size of the allowable error (α) for each comparison by the number of comparisons that are performed results in an overall α that does not exceed the desired limit.

In practical terms, the major differences between the various tests are the mathematical computations involved, the types of comparisons made

Table 27.3 Multiple comparison tests.

Fischer LSD
Bonferroni
Scheffé
Tukey
Newman–Keuls (also known as the Student–Newman–Keuls or SNK)
Duncan (also known as Duncan new multiple range)
Dunnett

among the data and the calculated probability levels established for each comparison. Thus, each test will indicate different probabilities and statistically significant differences between/among data items. This can be demonstrated by entering the same data into ProStat and performing each multiple comparison test in turn. It is beyond the scope of this book to discuss the mathematical bases of the varied multiple comparison tests but a few words about the most commonly used tests might be helpful. It should be stressed that statisticians do not generally agree as to which is the best procedure for identifying where differences lie in data sets.

Mathematically, the simplest multiple comparison procedure is *Fischer's LSD* (least significant difference) test. This test is the easiest one to perform manually but it is also the least conservative multiple comparison method.

The *Bonferroni's method* is also relatively simple to perform manually but because it compares every datum item to every other datum item, it tends to be overly conservative. The Bonferroni's method results in a true α that is substantially smaller than 0.05 when the test statistics are highly dependent and/or when many of the null hypotheses are false so that an unnecessarily high percentage of the true differences between datum items are not recognized.

The *Scheffé test* is especially suitable for multiple contrast tests such as those involving a null hypothesis that there is no difference between two samples. It is somewhat less conservative than the *Tukey HSD* (honestly significant difference) test.

The *Tukey test* is widely accepted and is one of the most conservative tests; it is very suitable when only pairwise comparisons are to be made. However, when many or all contrasts in a data set might be of interest, Scheffé's method is often preferred.

The *Newman–Keuls (or Student–Newman–Keuls) test* is similar to the Tukey test in that it determines differences between means but it is designed to calculate a different critical value for such differences. This results in different significance levels for rejecting the null hypothesis.

The *Duncan test* has a different theoretical basis from those of the Tukey and Newman–Keuls tests and uses a modified t statistic to compare sets of means. Duncan's test has been criticized as being too liberal by many statisticians although it is used quite frequently.

Another test that is sometimes used is *Dunnett's test*, which compares group means and is specifically designed for analyses in which all groups are compared to a single reference group. Dunnett's test analyses the null hypothesis that no group has a mean significantly different from the mean of the reference group.

Ideally, equal sample sizes should be used in multiple comparisons testing and most tests require normally distributed data. If the data are not normally distributed, performing the test procedures on the logarithms of the datum points can overcome this problem. Special procedures are available for data with inhomogeneous variances and for data with unequal N values.

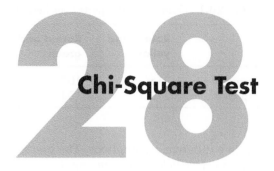

Chi-Square Test

The *chi-square test* (χ^2 test) is very useful for analyzing situations in which the researcher wants to determine whether a data sample conforms to a specified theoretical distribution, a method known as *goodness of fit* analysis. In other words, the procedure is used to test the difference between discrete distributions. There are, however, two ways of performing this analysis: (a) the sample distribution is compared with the expected distribution, and (b) two sample distributions are compared against each other.

Certain restrictions apply to using the χ^2 test. First, the test can only be performed on nominal scale data; that is, the data comprise counts of items or events in each of several classifications, for example, numbers of heads and tails when flipping a coin, etc. Second, there should be a precise statement of the null hypothesis being tested. In the coin example, the null hypothesis would be that when a coin is flipped 20 times, heads should occur 10 times.

The test procedure involves calculating the χ^2 statistic given by:

$$\chi^2 = \Sigma \frac{\left\{ (O - E)^2 \right\}}{E}$$

where O is the observed frequency of an event and E is the expected (theoretical) frequency of that event. This is a case (a) situation and a large χ^2 indicates that the null hypothesis (H_0: the observed distributions are drawn from the expected distribution) is unlikely.

This calculation, at least for simple comparisons, is easily performed using an Excel spreadsheet; however, tabulated values of the χ^2 distribution have to be consulted to determine the significance of the calculated χ^2 value.

Excel will perform a χ^2 test but it only returns the probability level without stating the χ^2 value. In contrast, ProStat presents the χ^2 value, the degrees of freedom and the probability, but the reader should be aware of the fact that the ProStat report actually presents two sets of data based

Table 28.1   Observed and expected numbers of peas in Mendel's heredity study.

	Round and yellow	Round and green	Wrinkled and yellow	Wrinkled and green
Observed	315	108	101	32
Expected	313	104	104	35

on two different assumptions. The first is that for data presented in two columns (see below), where one data column contains the observed values and the other contains the expected values—that is, a case (a) situation and the ProStat report for this calculation is labeled *one binned*. In the other situation, case (b), ProStat calculates χ^2 based on the assumption that the two columns are independent distributions. It should be noted that the χ^2 test in ProStat is found in the drop-down menu for nonparametric statistical tests.

As an example, consider Mendel's celebrated experiment with peas in which he counted the numbers of different pea types that grew. His theory was that the pea types should grow in accordance with a 9:3:3:1 ratio (Table 28.1).

Entering the data into an Excel spreadsheet and performing the χ^2 calculation produces the result shown in Table 28.2.

The calculated χ^2 value (0.510) is very small and from the χ^2 distribution table for $df = 3 (\chi^2_{0.05,3} = 7.81)$, it can be seen that Mendel's findings were in accord with his theory; that is, H_0 is accepted with a probability of $P < 0.95$ that this occurred by chance.

When this calculation is performed using the built-in subroutine in Excel, the data in Figure 28.1 is produced.

The data in Figure 28.1 are known as 4×2 *contingency table* since there are four rows ($h = 4$) and two columns ($k = 2$). The degrees of freedom (df) are given by multiplying ($h - 1$) by ($k - 1$); that is, $df = (4 - 1) \times (2 - 1) = 3$.

Table 28.2   Calculation of χ^2 in a spreadsheet.

	Round and yellow	Round and green	Wrinkled and yellow	Wrinkled and green
Observed	315	108	101	32
Expected	313	104	104	35
$(O - E)^2/E =$	0.013	0.154	0.087	0.257
$\chi^2 =$	0.510			

	Observed	Expected
Round, yellow	315	313
Round, green	108	104
Wrinkled, yellow	101	104
Wrinkled, green	32	35
$P =$	0.963	← ———— =CHITEST(b2:b4, c2:c4)

Figure 28.1 Calculation of the probability value for Mendel's study. (The Excel instruction is indicated in the figure.)

ProStat, performing the χ^2 test on the above data, produces the report shown in Figure 28.2.

Thus, all three approaches yield the same information although ProStat dispenses with the need for consulting the χ^2 distribution table.

In many situations, the expected outcome is unknown but can be estimated. As a hypothetical example, two treatments have been developed for treating acute periodontitis and were administered to 20 patients (Table 28.3).

This problem can be approached in two ways. In one approach, it could be estimated that 70% of patients will benefit from both treatments so that an observed versus expected table can be produced (Table 28.4).

```
Nonparametric statistics report

One binned data chi-square test:
        Observed value:        Observed
        Expected value:        Expected
        Degree of freedom:        3
        Chi-square:        0.470
        Probability:        0.925

Two binned data chi-square test:
        Data set 1:        Observed
        Data set 2:        Expected
        Degree of freedom:        3
        Chi-square:        0.239
        Probability:        0.971
```

Figure 28.2 ProStat χ^2 report for Mendel's study.

Table 28.3 Patient responses to periodontal treatments ($N = 20$ in each group).

	Treatment beneficial	No effect
Treatment A	15	5
Treatment B	13	7

Entering these data into ProStat yields the results shown in Figure 28.3. The ProStat program calculates the correct value of χ^2 with a probability of 0.92 for one binned data but because the program "sees" four rows of data, it calculates a $df = 3$.

The second approach is to enter the data into ProStat as shown in Table 28.5, the resulting χ^2 report is presented in Figure 28.4.

It can be seen from Figure 28.4 that only the two binned result should be accepted for the calculation of the χ^2 value because in the one binned calculation, the program assumed that the Treatment B data are expected values. Although the one binned calculation in Figure 28.3 and the two binned calculation in Figure 28.4 gave the same value of χ^2, the probabilities of significance were different. However, both approaches indicate that H_0 should be accepted since $P > 0.05$.

Chi-square tests are not limited to 2×2 data tables but data involving more than two columns cannot be processed with ProStat unless the data are in the form of Observed/Expected findings, where the expected findings are hypothesized or based upon an average for the whole data set.

Another factor in χ^2 testing is that the expected value in each cell should be ≥ 5. This problem was addressed by Yates, who suggested that those values in the tabulated data which exceeded expectation should be decreased by 0.5, whereas values that did not reach expectation should be increased by 0.5. An example of the Yates' correction is shown in Table 28.6. In this table, two groups of 50 patients each were administered

Table 28.4 Data from Table 28.3 expressed as observed/expected findings.

	Observed	Expected
Treatment A—benefit	15	14
Treatment B—benefit	13	14
Treatment A—no effect	5	6
Treatment B—no effect	7	6

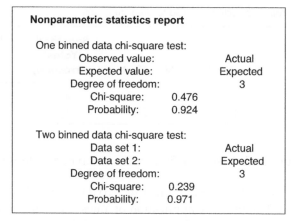

```
Nonparametric statistics report

One binned data chi-square test:
          Observed value:                Actual
          Expected value:                Expected
          Degree of freedom:                3
              Chi-square:      0.476
              Probability:     0.924

Two binned data chi-square test:
          Data set 1:                    Actual
          Data set 2:                    Expected
          Degree of freedom:                3
              Chi-square:      0.239
              Probability:     0.971
```

Figure 28.3 Chi-squared report in ProStat.

Table 28.5 Rearrangement of data from Table 28.3 for insertion into ProStat.

	Treatment A	**Treatment B**
Benefited	15	13
No effect	5	7

```
Nonparametric statistics report

One binned data chi-square test:
          Observed value:                Treatment A
          Expected value:                Treatment B
          Degree of freedom:                1
              Chi-square:      0.879
              Probability:     0.348

Two binned data chi-square test:
          Data set 1:                    Treatment A
          Data set 2:                    Treatment B
          Degree of freedom:                1
              Chi-square:      0.476
              Probability:     0.490
```

Figure 28.4 Chi-squared report in ProStat.

Table 28.6 Yates' correction applied to drug study data.

	Benefited	No effect	Benefited (Yates' correction)	No effect (Yates' correction)
Drug A	4	46	4.5	45.5
Drug B	8	42	7.5	42.5

different drugs and those benefiting were compared to those that registered no effect.

The χ^2 value for the original (uncorrected) data was 1.515 with a probability $P = 0.679$. Following application of Yates' correction, the χ^2 value decreases to 0.852 with a probability $P = 0.837$. In the present example, Yates' correction did not greatly affect the significance level but in cases where the χ^2 is close to statistical significance, then applying the correction can be an important safeguard against claiming unjustifiable significance.

Bartlett's Test

In Chapter 27, Figure 27.4, reference was made to *Bartlett's χ^2 test* for homogeneity of variance, a test to determine whether all samples came from populations with equal or homogeneous variances. The term for homogeneity of variances is *homoscedasticity* and its antonym is *heteroscedasticity*. In other words, Bartlett's test determines whether all sample variances estimate the same population variance. Some statistical tests, for example, analysis of variance, assume that variances are equal among groups or samples and the Bartlett's test can be used to verify that assumption. The computations involved in Bartlett's test are tedious when performed manually but ProStat calculates Bartlett's χ^2 value when performing multiple comparisons. In the cited example, Bartlett's $\chi^2 = 2.716$ ($P = 0.95$) and H_0 (all variances were homogeneous) can be accepted.

Bartlett's test, and the majority of other variance homogeneity tests, is adversely affected by non-normal populations and its power is markedly reduced. This affects the validity of its application in determining variance homogeneity in multisample comparisons among means of non-normal data.

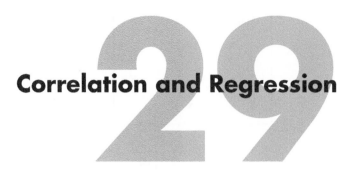

Correlation and Regression

In many situations, it is useful to assess the *degree of association* in a *bivariate* population (i.e., between two sets of data). Typical examples of associated variates (datum items) are height and weight, parental and child IQ scores, fluoride ingestion and dental caries, and so forth. Although examples of precise interrelationships are rare, a degree of association or *correlation* is quite common. The degree of correlation is expressed as the *coefficient of correlation* (R). If there is a perfect correlation between two variates ($R = 1$), whereas $R = 0$ when there is absolutely no correlation or association between the variates.

When data are plotted on a scattergram (see Figure 22.8), the data can be inspected for the degree of association (Figure 29.1).

Data in Figure 29.1a have no clear association and are non-correlated ($R = 0$), whereas there is a partial correlation ($0 < R < 1$) among the data in Figure 29.1b. The two variates in Figure 29.1c are closely correlated and $R \rightarrow 1$.

LINEAR REGRESSION

When data such as those in Table 29.1 are plotted as a scattergram and a trend line is inserted (Figure 29.2), it is immediately obvious that not only are the two variates, height and weight, closely correlated, but all data lie close to the *trend line*.

Since the trend line is linear, the relationship between the variates (X and Y) may be expressed by a linear equation: $Y = a + b \times X$, where a and b are constants. In this example, Y increases as X increases and there is a *positive* or direct correlation between X and Y. If Y decreases as X increases, the association between the two variates is said to be a negative

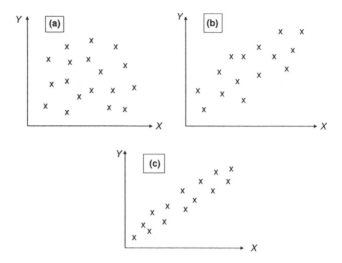

Figure 29.1 Data in (a) are noncorrelated, data in (b) are partially correlated, whereas data in (c) are closely correlated.

or an *inverse* correlation. It should be noted that there are many different types of trend lines and Excel will calculate and insert them directly into the scattergram from the drop-down Chart menu.

The trend line in Figure 29.2 is known as a linear regression line with the form $Y = a + b \times X$ and this equation can be used to predict values

Table 29.1 Heights and corresponding weights of 12 high school students.

Height (cm)	Weight (kg)
142.2	36.4
144.8	34.1
147.3	36.8
147.3	37.7
149.9	37.3
152.4	40.9
154.0	42.0
157.5	42.3
162.6	43.6
163.0	44.5
167.6	49.0
170.2	48.0

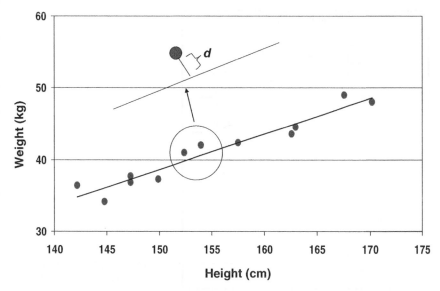

Figure 29.2 Scattergram of data in Table 29.1 with added trend line.

of Y for different X values, and vice versa, when the values of constants a and b are known.

As an aside, it should be noted that traits in one generation do not inevitably increase in succeeding generations. Thus, for example, whereas the children of tall parents are usually tall themselves, the grandchildren may be near average in height. The same trend is often seen with such characteristics as intelligence, artistic ability, musical talent etc. This behavior in succeeding generations is known as *regression to the mean*.

LEAST-SQUARES LINE

The *goodness of fit* of the trend line to the experimental data is given by the sum of the squares of the deviation of each point, shown as "d" in Figure 29.2. The fit of the trend line to the experimental data improves with smaller values of the sum of all the squared deviations, that is, fit improves as $\sum d^2 \to 0$, and the best fitting line is known as the *least-squares line* (LSL). The values of constants a and b can be calculated from the data using the following equations (note that N is the number of specimens):

$$a = \frac{(\Sigma Y) \times (\Sigma X^2) - (\Sigma X) \times (\Sigma XY)}{N \times \Sigma X^2 - (\Sigma X)^2}$$

	Height (cm)	Weight (kg)
	142.2	36.4
	144.8	34.1
	147.3	36.8
	147.3	37.7
	149.9	37.3
	152.4	40.9
	154.0	42.0
	157.5	42.3
	162.6	43.6
	163.0	44.5
	167.6	49.0
	170.2	48.0
Slope, b =	0.496	←———— =LINEST(C2:C13,B2:B13)
Intercept, a =	−35.721	←———— =INTERCEPT(C2:C13,B2:B13)

Figure 29.3 Calculation of the parameters a and b in the regression (least squares) line for the data in Table 29.1.

and

$$b = \frac{N \times \Sigma XY - (\Sigma X) \times (\Sigma Y)}{N \times \Sigma X^2 - (\Sigma X)^2}$$

The constant a is the intercept of the LSL with the ordinate or Y-axis and constant b is the slope of the LSL line. Fortunately, Excel will calculate these parameters, as shown in Figure 29.3, and the equation of the LSL or regression line for the data in Table 29.1 is:

$$Y = -35.721 + 0.496.X$$

or, student weight (kg) = (0.496 × student height) − 35.721 cm.

COEFFICIENT OF CORRELATION

The total variation of the Y data (student weights in the above example) is the sum of the squares of the deviations of the Y values from the mean Y value, $\overline{Y}$.

Total variation of $Y = \Sigma(Y - \overline{Y})^2$, which can be written as total variation of $Y = \Sigma(Y - Y_c)^2 + \Sigma(Y_c - \overline{Y})^2$, where Y_c is the value of y calculated for a given X from the regression line of Y on X.

Table 29.2 Correlation analysis for the data in Table 29.1.

	Correlation	
	Height (cm)	**Weight (kg)**
Height (cm)	1	
Weight (kg)	0.966	1

The first term, $\Sigma(Y - Y_c)^2$, is known to vary in a random manner and is called the random or *unexplained variation* of Y. The second term, $\Sigma(Y_c - \overline{Y})^2$, varies predictably and is known as the *explained variation* of Y. The ratio of the explained variation to the total variation of Y is known as the *coefficient of determination* (R^2), where $0 \leq R^2 \leq 1$. When $R^2 = 1$, there is no random variation of Y, and when $R^2 = 0$, all variation of Y is unexplained or completely random.

The square root of the coefficient of determination is known as the *coefficient of correlation* (R):

$$R = \sqrt{\frac{\text{explained variation}}{\text{total variation}}}$$

and since $0 \leq R^2 \leq 1$, R can have any value from -1 to $+1$, or $-1 \leq R \leq 1$.

The value of the coefficient of correlation (R) can be obtained with the *correlation analysis tool* under Excel's drop-down menu *Tools: Data analysis*. This analysis in the Excel spreadsheet for the data in Table 29.1 is presented as Table 29.2.

The analysis indicates that the correlation between student heights and weights is 0.966, that is, the two statistics are very closely correlated at approximately 97%.

STATISTICAL SIGNIFICANCE OF THE CORRELATION COEFFICIENT

Often, the researcher may wish to determine the statistical significance of the correlation coefficient (R). This can be performed manually by using the relationship:

$$t = \frac{t \times \sqrt{(N-2)}}{\sqrt{(1 - R^2)}}$$

Table 29.3 Regression analysis of data in Table 29.1 using Excel.

SUMMARY OUTPUT

Regression statistics

Multiple R	0.966
R^2	0.934
Adjusted R^2	0.927
Standard error	1.277
Observations	12

ANOVA

	df	SS	MS	F	Significance of F
Regression	1	230.132	230.132	141.136	3.21×10^{-7}
Residual	10	16.306	1.631		
Total	11	246.437			

	Coefficients	Standard error	t stat	P value	Lower 95%	Upper 95%	Lower 95.0%	Upper 95.0%
Intercept	−35.721	6.473	−5.519	0.000	−50.143	−21.298	−50.143	−21.298
Height (cm)	0.496	0.042	11.880	0.000	0.403	0.589	0.403	0.589

which has Student's t distribution for $N - 2$ degrees of freedom. The significance of the calculated value of R is then determined from the t distribution table.

Fortunately, the need to calculate manually the value of t and consult the t distribution table is obviated by using the *Regression Analysis* program within the Excel's *statistics data analysis tool box*. Following the prompts and entering the data from Table 29.1 yields the summary report shown in Table 29.3.

The regression analysis summary output from Excel provides a wealth of information, notably the values of the correlation coefficient ($R = 0.966$), the intercept ($a = -35.721$), the slope of the LSL ($b = 0.496$) together with the significances of the values of R, a, and b ($P < 0.001$). The summary output also provides the upper and lower confidence limits for the values of a and b. This regression analysis indicates that there is a very close correlation between the heights and weights of the students in the present example and that, statistically, the correlation is highly significant.

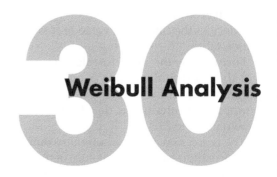

Weibull Analysis

Weibull analysis is a method for modeling data sets that allows various predictions to be made. It has been used for a variety of applications, including predicting product service life based on failure rate data, AIDS mortality rates, and earthquake probabilities. The analysis is based on the Weibull cumulative distribution function,

$$F(X) = 1 - e^{-[X/\alpha]^{\beta}}$$

where $F(X)$ is the Weibull distribution function for X, which for computational purposes (see below) is often transformed into a linear form:

$$Ln\left\{Ln\left[\frac{1}{1 - F(X)}\right]\right\} = \beta \times Ln\ X - \beta \times Ln\ \alpha$$

The transformed Weibull function resembles the equation for a straight line $(Y = a + b \times X)$ so that when a linear regression analysis is performed, the Weibull parameter β is given by the slope of the regression line. However, the Weibull parameter α must be calculated: $\alpha = \exp[-(\text{intercept}, a)/\beta]$. The values of the Weibull parameters must be known in order to perform a Weibull analysis.

As mentioned above, a common application of a Weibull analysis is in failure analysis and product service life predictions. In this application, the *Weibull shape parameter β* indicates whether the failure rate is increasing, decreasing, or remaining constant (Table 30.1).

Specialized software is available for performing Weibull analyses. Excel contains a Weibull program in its drop-down menu in the data analysis suite and, when the Weibull parameters are known, will provide probability information required for survival predictions (see below). Determination of the requisite Weibull parameters can be performed using the Excel spreadsheet as shown in the following example.

A manufacturer has two adhesive formulations for direct bonding of orthodontic brackets. The design specification is that the adhesives

Table 30.1   Failure behavior predicted by the Weibull shape parameter.

Value of the shape parameter	Trend in behavior
$\beta < 1.0$	Decreasing failure rate [failure during "burn-in" period]
$\beta = 1.0$	Constant failure rate
$\beta > 1.0$	Increasing failure rate [failure over time, material fatigue, or deterioration]

achieve shear bond strength (SBS) values of 15 MPa when bonding brackets to a standard substrate, bovine tooth enamel. Two sets of ten brackets were bonded to extracted, cleaned, and sanitized bovine teeth with the two adhesives and SBS testing was performed; the data are presented in Table 30.2 and Figure 30.1.

No statistically significant difference ($P > 0.05$) was found between the two data sets. Although there was no significant difference between the SBS values, a decision had to be made as to which adhesive might have the more reliable retention ability in clinical practice and the problem was addressed by means of a Weibull analysis.

The Weibull parameters α and β must be derived in order to perform a Weibull analysis and the procedure for this is shown for the Adhesive A specimens (Table 30.3).

Table 30.2   Shear bond strengths (SBS) for two orthodontic adhesives.

	Adhesive A	Adhesive B
	9.85	12.44
	11.92	13.56
	12.23	16.18
	13.38	16.54
	15.29	16.58
	16.38	17.34
	16.73	17.49
	17.29	17.57
	18.57	18.47
	19.46	18.54
Mean	15.11	16.47
S.Dev.	3.15	2.00
CofV, %	20.82	12.16

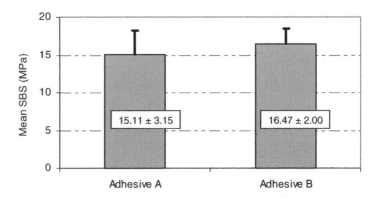

Figure 30.1 Mean shear bond strengths for two orthodontic adhesives (MPa).

PROCEDURE

1. Place SBS values in Column A and a rank is assigned to each datum item in Column B.
2. Calculate the median rank using Excel instruction: $= (A2 - 0.3)/(N + 0.4)$, where $N = 10$ for ten specimens. This calculation of the median rank (MR), that is, $MR = (j - 0.3)/(N + 0.4)$, where j is the datum item, is known as *Barnard's approximation*.
3. Calculate the value of $1/(1 -$ median rank) using Excel instruction: $= 1/(1 - C2)$
4. Calculate the natural logarithm of the natural logarithm of $1/(1 -$ median rank) using Excel instruction: *LN(LN(D2))*.

Table 30.3 Preparation of Adhesive A data for Weibull analysis.

SBS	Rank	Median ranks	1/(1 − median rank)	Ln(Ln(1/1 − median rank))	Ln(Adhesive A)
9.85	1	0.067	1.072	−2.664	2.287
11.92	2	0.163	1.195	−1.723	2.478
12.23	3	0.260	1.351	−1.202	2.504
13.38	4	0.356	1.552	−0.822	2.594
15.29	5	0.452	1.825	−0.509	2.727
16.38	6	0.548	2.213	−0.230	2.796
16.73	7	0.644	2.811	0.033	2.817
17.29	8	0.740	3.852	0.299	2.850
18.57	9	0.837	6.118	0.594	2.922
19.46	10	0.933	14.857	0.993	2.968

Table 30.4 Regression analysis of the Adhesive A data.

SUMMARY OUTPUT

Regression statistics

Multiple R	0.989
R^2	0.979
Adjusted R^2	0.976
Standard error	0.172
Observations	10

ANOVA

	df	SS	MS	F	Significance of F
Regression	1	10.952	10.952	368.289	0.000
Residual	8	0.238	0.030		
Total	9	11.190			

	Coefficients	Standard error	t stat	P value
Intercept	−14.025	0.706	−19.875	0.000
Ln(Adhesive A)	5.011	0.261	19.191	0.000
$\beta =$	**5.011**			
$\alpha =$	**16.425**			

Weibull α is calculated using the instruction: = EXP(−B16/B17). In this example, $\alpha = \exp\,[14.025 \div 5.011] = 16.425$.

5. Calculate the natural logarithm of the datum item using Excel instruction: = $LN(A2)$.
6. Copy C2:F2 to rows C3 to C11.

Column E contains the Y values and Column F contains the X values for the regression equation ($Y = \alpha + \beta \times X$). A regression analysis can now be performed on the data using Column E as the Y values and Column F as the X values. The Weibull parameters α and β are calculated from the regression summary report (Table 30.4).

Performing the same calculation for the Adhesive B data yields the Weibull parameters shown in Table 30.5.

Since $\beta > 1$ for the two sets of data, both types of adhesive will eventually fail under bond strength testing. The Weibull characteristic α is a measure of the spread in the data distribution and, on theoretical

Table 30.5 Weibull parameters for orthodontic adhesive SBS data.

	Adhesive A	**Adhesive B**
Weibull (β)	5.011	8.144
Weibull (α)	16.425	17.435

grounds and regardless of the value of β, $\alpha =$ the SBS at which 63.2% of the Adhesive A specimens have a shear bond strength $\leq$ 16.4 MPa and 36.8% of specimens have an SBS $\geq$ 16.4 MPa. Similarly, for Adhesive B, approximately 63% specimens will have an SBS $\leq$ 17.4 MPa and 37% have an SBS $\geq$ 17.4 MPa.

The required SBS value was 15 MPa and it is possible to calculate a reliability value (R_X) for the two adhesives using the relationship:

$$R_X = e^{-(X/\alpha)^\beta},$$

where X is the required value of SBS. Accordingly,

$$\text{Adhesive A}: R_{15} = e^{-(15/16 \cdot 425)^{5.011}} = 0.530$$

and

$$\text{Adhesive B}: R_{15} = e^{-(15/17 \cdot 435)^{8.144}} = 0.745$$

and the Weibull analysis predicts that 53% of Adhesive A and 75% of Adhesive B specimens will achieve SBS values $\geq$ 15 MPa. If the SBS requirement is decreased to 14 MPa, the reliability estimates increase:

$$\text{Adhesive A}: R_{14} = e^{-(14/16 \cdot 425)^{5.011}} = 0.638$$

and

$$\text{Adhesive B}: R_{14} = e^{-(14/17 \cdot 435)^{8.144}} = 0.846.$$

It is possible to construct a *survival probability table* (Table 30.6) based on the Weibull parameters and by means of the Weibull analytical tool in the Excel drop-down *Data Analysis Tool Box*. The Excel instruction to calculate the SBS probability is $= WEIBULL(A7,\$B\$3,\$B\$4,True)$, in which A7 refers to the SBS value, $\$B\$3$ is the value of α, and $\$B\$4$ is the value of β. The Excel instruction *True* indicates that the Weibull program should calculate the cumulative distribution function. If *False* is used in the instruction, then the Weibull program returns the probability density function. The reliability is given by $1 - probability$ and the number of specimens is $100 \times the\ reliability$.

Table 30.6 Survival table for Adhesive A data.

Adhesive A

β (Shape parameter):   5.011
α (Characteristic):   16.425

SBS	SBS probability	Reliability	Specimens (%)
10	0.0798	0.9202	92.0
11	0.1255	0.8745	87.4
12	0.1874	0.8126	81.3
13	0.2664	0.7336	73.4
14	0.3618	0.6382	63.8
15	*0.4699*	*0.5301*	*53.0*
16	0.5840	0.4160	41.6
17	0.6953	0.3047	30.5
18	0.7945	0.2055	20.5
19	0.8744	0.1256	12.6
20	0.9316	0.0684	6.8

The values for specification SBS of 15 MPa are in italics.

A *reliability* table (Table 30.7) can also be constructed based on the relationship given above. In this table, the Excel instruction: $= \alpha*(-LN(A2)^{\wedge}(1/\beta))$ calculates the SBS value that each adhesive will achieve at the specified reliability value in Column A.

These data can be presented in graphical form by calculating as indicated above the probabilities and reliabilities at each SBS values for the two adhesives (Table 30.8).

Table 30.7 Reliability table for SBS values.

	SBS		
Reliability	Adhesive A	Adhesive B	Specimens (%)
0.01	22	20	1
0.05	20	19	5
0.10	19	18	10
0.25	18	17	25
0.50	15	15	50
0.75	13	14	75
0.90	10	12	90

Table 30.8 Survival table for Adhesive A and Adhesive B data.

	Adhesive A		Adhesive B	
SBS	**Probability**	**Reliability**	**Probability**	**Reliability**
1	0.0000	1.0000	0.0000	1.0000
2	0.0000	1.0000	0.0000	1.0000
3	0.0002	0.9998	0.0000	1.0000
4	0.0008	0.9992	0.0000	1.0000
5	0.0026	0.9974	0.0000	1.0000
6	0.0064	0.9936	0.0002	0.9998
7	0.0138	0.9862	0.0006	0.9994
8	0.0268	0.9732	0.0018	0.9982
9	0.0479	0.9521	0.0046	0.9954
10	0.0798	0.9202	0.0108	0.9892
11	0.1255	0.8745	0.0232	0.9768
12	0.1874	0.8126	0.0466	0.9534
13	0.2664	0.7336	0.0875	0.9125
14	0.3618	0.6382	0.1542	0.8458
15	0.4699	0.5301	0.2545	0.7455
16	0.5840	0.4160	0.3915	0.6085
17	0.6953	0.3047	0.5569	0.4431
18	0.7945	0.2055	0.7265	0.2735
19	0.8744	0.1256	0.8665	0.1335
20	0.9316	0.0684	0.9530	0.0470

Thereafter, using the *Chart Wizard* in Excel, plotting the adhesive reliabilities against the corresponding SBS values produces a *survival graph* (Figure 30.2).

The survival graph clearly indicates that Adhesive B exhibits a better performance than Adhesive A, a prediction that could not be made from a statistical analysis such as ANOVA. In particular, ANOVA indicated that there was no statistically significant difference in SBS values for the two adhesives. Further, it can be seen from the survival table (Table 30.8) that only 53% of orthodontic brackets bonded with Adhesive A are predicted to achieve the specified SBS of 15 MPa compared to 75% of orthodontic brackets bonded with Adhesive B.

It is possible to plot on one graph the survival predictions for several entities, thereby facilitating a direct and readily apparent comparison of their performances. An example is shown in Figure 30.3.

It can be seen immediately that Adhesive D is superior to the other three adhesives and, further, that Adhesive C exhibits unacceptable shear bond strengths for orthodontic brackets.

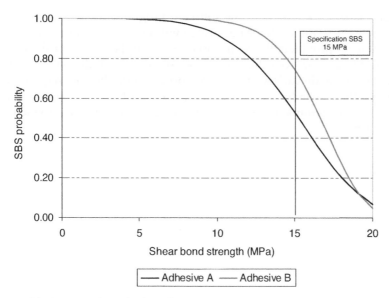

Figure 30.2 Survival graphs for Adhesives A and B.

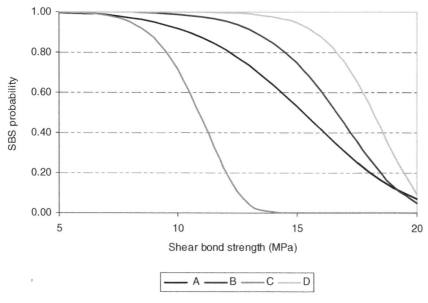

Figure 30.3 Survival graphs for four orthodontic adhesives.

Specialized Weibull analysis software programs are available but the requisite calculations can be performed within the Excel spreadsheet if the instructions provided above are used as a template for the calculations. It should be clear from the above example that Weibull analyses can be applied to a wide variety of research applications. The only requirements are that the researcher is careful when selecting the question to be asked as well as the parameter to be analyzed when entering data into the Excel spreadsheet.

Ranking Tests

Measurements must be made with the greatest possible precision so that the researcher can be confident that differences between sets of data are real differences and not due to imprecision of the measuring technique. Unfortunately, in the biological and sociological sciences, performing exact or precise measurements are often very difficult and perhaps even impossible. When data comprise opinions or assessments rather than numerical values, those individual datum items are known as *nonparametric statistics*.

Every dentist, when examining a patient, will make a chart entry regarding oral hygiene. It is easy for dentists to recognize a patient with "excellent" oral hygiene because there is a complete absence of plaque and calculus, whereas a patient with "poor" oral hygiene will have significant plaque/calculus deposits. Distinguishing between "excellent" and "poor" oral hygiene is straightforward but how does the clinician grade intermediate levels of oral hygiene? The same problem arises with other issues such as gingival hyperplasia, periodontal inflammation as well as determining practitioner competence. Identifying the extremes is quite simple but categorizing the intermediate stages is challenging.

In certain cases, it is possible to assign a numeric value or to score clinical observations. The Gingival index (GI) of Loe and Silness, for example, scores the amount of gingivitis on a scale of 0–3 according to defined criteria for no inflammation (0), slight inflammation (1), moderate inflammation (2), and severe inflammation (3). The scores for different areas of the mouth are then summed to give a total mouth score. Although the GI is very useful for evaluating the success/failure of periodontal treatment regimens, it still requires grading of oral conditions by the clinician. Various ranking tests have been developed to address such cases of nonparametric statistics.

Table 31.1   Ratings of patient oral hygiene by two periodontists.

Patient:	A	B	C	D	E	F	G	H	I	J
Periodontist (X)	2	1	3	4	6	5	8	10	7	9
Periodontist (Y)	1	2	3	6	5	7	6	10	9	8
Rank difference ($d = (Y-X)$)	−1	1	0	2	−1	2	−2	0	2	−1
Square of differences (d^2)	1	1	0	4	1	4	4	0	4	1

SPEARMAN'S RANK CORRELATION

Spearman's rank correlation is analogous to the coefficient of correlation used for parametric data and is a method of correlating the series of rankings or ranking scores obtained by one examiner with the rankings obtained by another examiner. As an example, consider two experienced periodontists each examining the same ten patients and ranking the patients from 0 to 10 on the basis of their perceived oral hygiene efficiency. Ideally, the two clinicians will score the same patient identically but, in reality, that seldom happens. The findings of the hypothetical periodontists are shown in Table 31.1 together with the rank difference d (the difference in patient scores by the examiners) and the value of d^2.

Spearman's rank correlation R_s is calculated using the formula:

$$R_s = 1 - \frac{6 \times \Sigma d^2}{N^3 - N}$$

where N is the number specimens (patients) and Σd^2 is the sum of the squares of the differences between periodontist ratings. In this example, $N = 10$ and $\Sigma d^2 = 20$ so that

$$R_s = 1 - \frac{6 \times 20}{1000 - 10} = 1 - \frac{120}{990} = 0.88$$

If the two rankings had been identical, the rank difference would be 0 and $R_s = 1$ because there would be perfect correlation between the two examiners. With greater disagreement between the examiners, $R_s \rightarrow -1$ so that the value of R_s will range from −1 (complete disagreement) to +1 (complete agreement). In the present example, the examiners agreed completely about only two patients (C and H) but, nevertheless, there was an 88% agreement between the two examiners ($R_s = 0.88$).

The significance of this correlation can be tested using Student's t distribution as discussed in Chapter 13 for the correlation coefficient of parametric data:

$$t = R_s \times \sqrt{\frac{N-2}{1-R_s^2}} = 0.88 \times \sqrt{\frac{8}{1-0.77}} = 5.190$$

From the t distribution table, $t = 5.041$ at $df = 8$ at the 0.001 level of probability so that it can be concluded that there was no statistically significant difference in patient grading by the two periodontists ($P < 0.001$).

A variety of statistical evaluation procedures are available for testing nonparametric data, two of the most widely used being the *Wilcoxon matched-pairs signed-rank test* and the *Mann–Whitney U test*. Neither test uses the actual measurements; instead, they use the ranks of the data which have been ordered from the lowest to the highest (or vice versa). This approach is used in many other nonparameter procedures.

WILCOXON MATCHED-PAIRS SIGNED-RANK TEST

Researchers often want to establish whether one treatment is superior to another when used for two groups of patients. However, in order to do so, the two patient groups must be very similar at the start of the treatment, that is, at base line; otherwise any observed differences might be due to differences within the groups rather than those due to the applied treatments. The effects arising from extraneous differences between the groups can be eliminated by using related samples in the project. Ideally, this is achieved by using several pairs of identical twins, with one twin assigned to one test group and the other to the alternative group so that the two groups are composed of very closely "matched pairs." Alternatively, a series of individuals can be used with each individual being provided with both treatments at different times so that, in effect, one is again looking at matched pairs. The *Wilcoxon matched-pairs signed-rank test* can then be used to determine the significance of any differences in treatments.

It is perhaps simplest to show what calculations are performed in the Wilcoxon test by means of an example. In this case, GI scores were assessed for a group of ten patients prior to and 3 months after oral hygiene instruction (Table 31.2).

In Table 31.2, Columns 1 and 2 indicate the GI scores pre- and postoral hygiene instruction, and Column 3 shows the differences in the scores.

In Column 4, the differences are ranked in increasing order of magnitude; those patients who show no difference between *pre-* versus *post-Tx* scores are eliminated in this ranking. Where there are identical or *tied* observations (patients A and I), each is given the average of the ranks they would have had if no ties had occurred.

Table 31.2 Pre- and posttreatment Gingival index scores and the ranking of differences.

Column:	1	2	3	4	5
Patient	Initial GI score	Post-Tx score	Difference	Rank of difference	Ranks with positive sign
A	11	4	7	7.5	7.5
B	12	6	6	6	6
C	24	10	14	9	9
D	9	10	−1	1	
E	7	7	0		
F	10	7	3	3	3
G	13	9	4	4	4
H	3	5	−2	2	
I	24	17	7	7.5	7.5
J	17	12	5	5	5
Sum:	130	87	43	$W =$	42

Initial GI score is the pre-treatment Gingival index score and Post-Tx is the posttreatment Gingival index score.

Column 5 shows the ranks with the more frequent sign, which in this case are patients showing a decrease in the GI score.

The sum of the ranks is the W *score* and in this example, $W = 42$. The significance of this value of W can be determined by consulting tabulated values of critical values of W at $N = 8$, where N is the total specimen count $(10 - 2)$. In the present example, based on the value of W, there is a statistically significant difference between the pre- and posttreatment GI scores.

The calculations for the Wilcoxon matched-pairs signed-rank test can be performed manually but it is much more convenient, and faster, to perform a Wilcoxon signed-rank test using ProStat. For this, the data are entered into the ProStat spreadsheet and then, under the drop-down box for *Statistics*, the *nonparametric/Wilcoxon signed-rank* command is selected. This brings up the *Wilcoxon signed-rank* dialog box into which are entered the two data columns to be tested. ProStat calculates the difference between the two samples and ranks the difference in increasing order of absolute value. Then ProStat obtains the test statistic W by summing the rank for differences with a positive sign and then calculates the *z-score* (see Chapter 21) for W and, based on the sample size, calculates the probability for a difference between the two groups (Figure 31.1).

The probability values indicate a significant difference of the median in the two samples and signaling that there is a statistically significant

```
┌─────────────────────────────────────────────────────┐
│                                                       │
│   The ProStat Wilcoxon signed-rank test report        │
│                                                       │
│   For columns pre-Tx–Post-Tx                          │
│   Wilcoxon signed-rank test result:                   │
│                 W value:            42                │
│                 Z value:            –2.3102           │
│          One-tailed probability:    0.0104            │
│          Two-tailed probability:    0.0209            │
│                                                       │
└─────────────────────────────────────────────────────┘
```

Figure 31.1   ProStat Wilcoxon signed-rank test report for data in Table 31.2.

difference between the groups. Based on this study, the conclusion may be drawn that oral hygiene instruction will reduce patient GI scores.

MANN–WHITNEY U TEST

The Mann–Whitney U test is a ranking test that is similar to the Wilcoxon rank-sum test; however, it is designed to be used when paired differences are unattainable; it is somewhat more powerful because the test can handle unequal-sized samples. In the Wilcoxon test, the combined samples are ranked in increasing order and the sum of ranks for the two samples is determined separately. In contrast, the test statistic U in the Mann–Whitney test is defined as the smaller of

$$U = N_1 N_2 + \frac{N_1(N_1 + 1)}{2} - R_1 \text{ or } U' = N_1 N_2 - U$$

where N_1 is the smaller sample size, N_2 is the larger sample size, and R_1 is the rank-sum of the smaller sample. When the sample size is large (i.e., $N_1 + N_2 > 20$), U is approximately normally distributed and a z-score can be calculated using:

$$z = (U - \mu_U)/\sigma_U = [U - \tfrac{1}{2} \times (N_1 \times N_2)]/\sqrt{\frac{(N_1 \times N_2) \times (N_1 + N_2 + 1)}{12}}$$

where   mean $\mu_U = \tfrac{1}{2} \times (N_1 N_2)$ and   standard   deviation $\sigma_U = \sqrt{\frac{(N_1 \times N_2) \times (N_1 + N_2 + 1)}{12}}$

The Mann–Whitney test is best illustrated by an example. A group of 20 people ($N_1 = 9$ males and $N_2 = 11$ females) have volunteered for a new treatment for gingivitis. The researcher needs to be assured that the base line GI scores are the same for both groups before including them in the study. The base line GI scores are shown in Table 31.3.

Parametric statistical analysis indicates that there is no difference ($P < 0.05$) between the two groups but these scores are not numerical

Table 31.3 Base line GI scores for male and female patients.

	Men	Women
	2	4
	6	5
	10	7
	11	9
	12	11
	13	12
	14	14
	19	15
	20	16
		17
		18
Mean	11.9	11.6
S.Dev	5.7	4.9

because they are based upon a grading scale rather than physical measurements. Accordingly, the use of parametric analysis is invalid. Instead the Mann–Whitney U test should be used to compare these two independent samples. The procedure is as follows.

First, the two sets of scores are ranked (Table 31.4).

The lowest score in either of the groups is given rank 1, the second lowest score is rank 2, etc. Again, if identical scores are found in both groups, that is, *tied* scores, the rank assigned to each of the tied scores is the mean of the ranks that would have been assigned to these scores if they had not been tied. Substituting the values for N_1 (9), N_2 (11), and R_1 (95.5) into the expression for U, one obtains:

$$U = N_1 N_2 + \frac{N_1(N_1 + 1)}{2} - R_1 = 48.5 \quad \text{and} \quad U' = N_1 N_2 - U = 50.5$$

Consulting the tabulated values of the critical values of U for N_1 (9) and N_2 (11) at the 0.05 level of significance in a two-tailed test, the critical value is $U_{0.05(2),9,11} = 76$. Since the calculated value of U is 48.5, the null hypothesis (H_0: no difference between the two groups) can be accepted.

The same computation can be performed in ProStat. The data are entered into the ProStat spreadsheet and then, under the drop-down box for *Statistics*, the *nonparametric/Mann–Whitney test* command is selected. This brings up the *Mann–Whitney test* dialog box into which are entered the two data columns to be tested. ProStat will rank the combined samples in increasing order and then find the sum of ranks for the two samples

Table 31.4 Ranked GI scores for male and female patients.

GI scores		Ranks	
Men	**Women**	**Men**	**Women**
2	4	1	2
6	5	4	3
10	7	7	5
11	9	8.5	6
12	11	10.5	8.5
13	12	12	10.5
14	14	13.5	13.5
19	15	19	15
20	16	20	16
	17		17
	18		18
Sum of ranks			
R_1 (males)		95.5	
R_2 (females)			114.5

separately. ProStat then calculates the corresponding Z value and also calculates one-tailed and two-tailed probabilities (Figure 31.2).

The Mann–Whitney test can also be used for ordinal data, such as examination or class grades where students have been awarded A, B, C, etc., grades. In this case, however, ProStat cannot perform the computation and ranking, and calculation of the value of U must be performed manually.

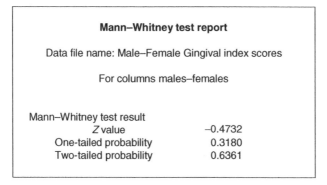

Mann–Whitney test report

Data file name: Male–Female Gingival index scores

For columns males–females

Mann–Whitney test result
Z value	–0.4732
One-tailed probability	0.3180
Two-tailed probability	0.6361

Figure 31.2 ProStat Mann–Whitney test report for data in Table 31.3.

There are a number of nonparametric statistical tests available for data analysis, each having certain advantages and disadvantages. There is little need within the context of this book to delve deeply into every possible nonparametric statistical test. Further information, however, is available in the monographs cited in the Appendix.

Appendix—Further Reading

It was stated in Chapter 17 that it is virtually impossible to write an acceptable dissertation or achieve publication of a manuscript in a reputable journal if the presented data have not been subjected to statistical analysis. The corollary of this statement is that the researcher should have a grasp of statistics and statistical analysis in order to perform a research study and successfully interpret the significance of the resulting data. Part II of this book is designed to provide researchers with the basics of statistical theory and analysis but this concise introduction, however useful, cannot replace formal courses, interactions with biomedical statisticians or careful study of the myriad books and monographs within this area. On the other hand, by providing the reader with a guide to the information that can be derived from inspection and examination of the data, it should be possible to undertake a variety of statistical tests that permit the researcher to draw valid and substantiated conclusions. Complex analyses, understandably, are beyond the scope of this book but in many situations, the information provided here should prove to be helpful to the researcher.

There are literally hundreds of monographs devoted to virtually every aspect of statistics and statistical analysis. Further, these books are pitched at every level from the very basic to highly complex treatments and are directed at almost every aspect of human endeavor requiring statistical analysis. Additionally, compilations of statistical tables (and graphs) that were mentioned in the text are available as stand-alone volumes as well as in appendices to many of the standard texts.

It would be nearly impossible to list every available book on statistical methods and analysis. However, a sampling of the plethora of available works is presented here. Many of these monographs, as mentioned above, contain compilations of the statistical tables required for determining statistical significance.

These monographs should be consulted by readers requiring further information on any of the topics discussed in the present book.

A. Indrayan. *Medical Biostatistics*. Chapman & Hall, London, UK (2007).

A. Petrie and C. Sabin. *Medical Statistics at a Glance*. Blackwell, Ames, IA (2005).

D. A. Lind. *Basic Statistics Using Excel for Office XP*, 12th edn. McGraw-Hill, New York (2005).

J. H. Zar. *Biostatistical Analysis*, 4th edn. Prentice-Hall, Upper Saddle River, NJ (1999).

J. Kim and R. Dailey. *Biostatistics in Oral Healthcare*. Wiley-Blackwell, Ames, IA (2007).

J. W. Kuzma and S. Bohnenblust. *Basic Statistics for the Health Sciences*, 5th edn. McGraw-Hill, New York (2005).

L. M. Sullivan. *Essentials of Biostatistics in Public Health*. Jones & Bartlett, Sudbury, MA (2008).

M. F. Triola, M. Triola, and M. M. Triola. *Biostatistics for the Biological and Health Sciences*. Addison-Wesley, Reading, MA (2005).

M. R Spiegel, J. J. Schiller, and R. A. Srinivasan. *Schaum's Outline of Probability and Statistics*, 3rd edn. McGraw-Hill, New York (2009).

R. C. Blair and R. A. Taylor. *Biostatistics for the Health Sciences*. Prentice Hall, Upper Saddle River, NJ (2007).

S. Siegel and N. J. Castellan Jr. *Nonparametric Statistics for the Behavioral Sciences*. McGraw-Hill, New York (1988).

Index

Printed and bound by CPI Group (UK) Ltd, Croydon, CR0 4YY

Printed and bound by CPI Group (UK) Ltd, Croydon, CR0 4YY

27/10/2024

14580240-0001